BIOETHICS
IN A
LIBERAL SOCIETY

BIOETHICS
IN A LIBERAL SOCIETY

THE POLITICAL FRAMEWORK
OF BIOETHICS DECISION MAKING

Thomas May

Associate Professor and Director of Graduate Studies in Bioethics
Center for the Study of Bioethics, Medical College of Wisconsin
Milwaukee, Wisconsin

The Johns Hopkins University Press
Baltimore and London

© 2002 The Johns Hopkins University Press
All rights reserved. Published 2002
Printed in the United States of America on acid-free paper
2 4 6 8 9 7 5 3 1

The Johns Hopkins University Press
2715 North Charles Street
Baltimore, Maryland 21218-4363
www.press.jhu.edu

Library of Congress Cataloging-in-Publication Data
May, Thomas, 1964–
    Bioethics in a liberal society : the political framework of
bioethics decision making / Thomas May
        p. ; cm.
Includes bibliographical references and index.
    ISBN 0-8018-6802-5 (hardcover : alk. paper)
1. Medical ethics. 2. Bioethics. 3. Liberalism.
    [DNLM: 1. Bioethics. 2. Patient Advocacy. 3. Decision
Making. 4. Professional Autonomy. W 85 M467b 2002]
I. Title.
    R724 .M278 2002
    174'.2—dc21

2001001335

A catalog record for this book is available from the British Library.

CONTENTS

PREFACE

THROUGHOUT THIS BOOK, I examine the rights and obligations that result from a liberal society's attempt to "balance" the autonomy of different individuals interacting in a common social setting. Along the way, I explore how a liberal perspective on autonomy and patient rights should shape our understanding of competency, advance directives, and the rights of both patients and health care providers.

Part I focuses on patient autonomy and the associated political rights, as well as the limits to patients' rights and the justification for those limits. Chapter 1 is an introduction to the issues and concepts in liberal political philosophy that serve as a framework for the book. In chapter 2, I examine why "patient autonomy" has come to assume such a prominent role in contemporary medicine and bioethics. Using the liberal framework, I consider how rights attached to patient autonomy result in the protection of individual judgment, including the right to make poor, or at times even "wrong," decisions. This right is mitigated, however, by the "harm principle," which allows certain public health exceptions to a patient's right to refuse treatment.

The liberal framework reserves a role in decision making for individual judgment. This role, however, presupposes certain capacities for making judgments and assuming responsibility. In chapter 3, I discuss these capacities and how they ground our judgment of a person's competence. In a liberal society we understand "competence" as denoting the eligibility to assume the role of autonomous decision making. Because in such a society this role allows individuals to adopt the values that will shape their lives and rejects a privileged point of view by which the merit of an individual's decision might be judged, our understanding of competence should be limited to a person's ability to direct her life in the context of the world around her.

When individuals are unable to fill the role reserved for individual judgment by a liberal constitutional society there results a "void" in decision making. This void creates problematic cases, and I end chapter 3 by discussing society's attempt to approach these circumstances as best we can, within a system specifically designed for persons who possess the capacity for autonomy. Included in this analysis is an examination of our approach to medical decision making for minors, individuals with severe mental handicaps, and persons with mental disorders.

Perhaps the most important mechanism we turn to when individuals are not able to make decisions for themselves is an advance directive, which is the focus of chapter 4. I examine how advance directives differ from active judgments and the implications of this for the ability of advance directives to stand in for individual judgment. Through this, we can understand the limitations placed on the application of advance directives and why these limitations differ among the various forms an advance directive might take, and we can identify concerns we should be conscious of when decisions are made using an advance directive.

Part II focuses on professional conscience and protection of the health care professional's autonomy-rights in the provider-patient relationship (as well as the professional obligations to which this relationship gives rise). The most striking professional obligation that mitigates the professional's autonomy is to respect the role of patient autonomy and informed consent in developing a treatment plan. This obligation partially modifies the professional's autonomy in his role as a health care provider.

Given the strong obligation to respect patient autonomy and informed consent, does any role remain in political liberalism for the concept of beneficence? In chapter 5, I argue that beneficence is important to our understanding of a minimal duty to aid or treat, within a professional-patient relationship. By examining society's (as well as the health care profession's) view of the responsibilities attached to the role of "health care professional," I explain a minimal duty to aid or treat through the obligation of nonabandonment, which is consistent with the liberal framework.

In chapter 6, I return to the balance of autonomy interests, which is what motivates a liberal society's focus on individual rights. I focus on the limits of liberal rights in requiring the participation of others in the pursuit of aims that an individual might adopt. These limits are reflected in our recognition of professional rights of conscience, and they shape our understanding of these rights in terms of the basis on which a right of conscience might be exercised.

Finally, in chapter 7, I examine the role of health care ethics committees and ethics consultants in a liberal context. Although in most areas of social life the protection of autonomy requires only a "hands-off" approach coupled with the concept of tolerance, patients in a clinical setting are particularly vulnerable. Thus, mechanisms designed to ensure that patient autonomy will be respected are called for. It is this role that health care ethics committees and consultants should strive to fill.

Throughout this book, I am concerned with the social interaction of individuals within the health care setting. I focus, then, on the rights and obligations of *individuals* interacting in such a setting, rather than on broader social policy questions concerning, for example, distributive justice. By examining the rights and obligations recognized by our political system, we identify an established set of boundaries for the application of personal moral beliefs, allowing the fundamental relevance of political philosophy for the most basic concepts of bioethics to emerge. Although substantive moral discussions about issues in bioethics are useful for individuals thinking about their personal convictions, any bioethics that fails to take seriously the political limits for the application of these moral beliefs risks becoming irrelevant to practice. Perhaps the unique feature of this book, is the emphasis it places on the relevance of *political philosophy* for day-to-day *clinical* decision making in bioethics.

ACKNOWLEDGMENTS

MANY PEOPLE CONTRIBUTED to the completion of this project. I would like to thank in particular Mark Aulisio, Jana Craig, and John Tomkowiak for comments and discussions that greatly improved the arguments in this book, and Laura Dillon and LaVar Matthews for their help in preparing the manuscript. The editorial help of Julie McCarthy at the Johns Hopkins University Press was particularly valuable. I would also like to thank my parents, Jerrold and Carol May, for their support in my career. Finally, I am grateful to the editors of several journals, in which some of the arguments and materials in this book have appeared: "Reassessing the Reliability of Advance Directives," *Cambridge Quarterly of Healthcare Ethics* 6, no. 3 (1997): 325–38; "Assessing Competency without Judging Merit," *Journal of Clinical Ethics* 9, no. 3 (1998): 247–57; "Bioethics in a Liberal Society," *International Journal of Applied Philosophy* 13, no. 1 (1999): 1–19; and "Rights of Conscience in Health Care," *Social Theory and Practice* 27, no. 1 (2001): 111–28.

BIOETHICS
IN A
LIBERAL SOCIETY

1

INTRODUCTION
The Liberal Framework

DEVELOPMENTS IN MEDICAL TECHNOLOGY offer tremendous advantages in many very important areas of life. But in making available treatment options that did not previously exist, these developments can infringe on other very important areas of life in ways once unfathomable. Blood transfusions, which offer medical benefits to certain patients, pose to persons with particular religious beliefs a threat that did not arise before the development of this technology. Treatment options such as chemotherapy offer potential benefits, but they also have potential side effects that might threaten a patient's dignity in ways that other treatment options would not. And our ability to continually extend biological life raises questions about whether simply extending life is our goal, or whether a longer life is a valid aim only when a patient considers his or her life to be of a quality worth living.

Judgment of the good by which "appropriate" treatment might be assessed, then, becomes a significant issue. There are many alternative frameworks by which this assessment might be made, as illustrated in a simplistic way by the examples mentioned above—the tension between extending biological life and quality of life or the use of blood products. Because medicine is, by nature, a social practice (involving the interaction, at a minimum, of patient and provider), the question arises: When the assessments of "better" from competing perspectives conflict, which values, or whose values, should frame the assessment that decides "better," or even "appropriate," treatment?

Understood in this way, the ethical questions surrounding the assessment of treatment become in large part political: Is there a privileged perspective that allows one individual's views to take precedence? If not, how do we determine which perspective assumes priority? These are not questions about the ultimate moral worth of a particular perspective, but rather are political questions concerning how to adjudicate between competing frameworks for assessing "the good."

In a liberal society, the answers to these questions depend on the individual and on the values that shape and give meaning to that individual's life. Liberal societies reject advocacy of substantive value systems at a social level in favor of a social system that defines value as determined, in substance or content, by individuals living in that society. In this, a plurality of values coexist, and no one of these, for social purposes, is given a privileged position.

Although rejection of a "privileged" perspective on the good often results in liberalism being associated with moral skepticism (see G. Dworkin 1974), and although moral skepticism is surely one foundation on which a liberal state might be adopted, liberalism does not require moral skepticism as a foundation (see Gray 1986). Indeed, such competing theories as those offered by John Rawls and utilitarianism emphasize the role of individual judgment and hardly need subscribe to a moral skepticism. The core idea of liberalism is that the individual is held to be the seat of moral judgment (see Hall and Ikenberry 1989), and this requires only that one recognize a diversity of views concerning moral questions, opting for a political structure that remains neutral among these, regardless whether one (or even more) of these is correct.

John Rawls (1971) takes the priority of "the right" over "the good" to be a starting point for his theory of justice, developing a political framework that he takes to embody a Kantian respect for autonomy. In emphasizing the priority of "the right," Rawls's theory of justice does not presuppose a privileged conception of the good but attempts to provide a political framework in the context of the good as understood through reference to the judgment of individuals.

John Stuart Mill (1956), a utilitarian, appealed to the importance of autonomy not because the right assumes priority over the good but rather because utility is served by allowing each individual to construct her own life plan. For Mill, the good consists of human "happiness," and this calls for maximizing the aggregate happiness of individuals living in a society. By

allowing individuals to construct their own life plans, their happiness is max-
imized. Although people may at times make poor decisions, the individual,
Mill argues, is in the best position to judge her own good.

This concern to respect individual judgment leads to a position of tolerance in social policy. A utilitarian argument for liberal tolerance of religious
moral perspectives relies on the idea that "even if the state could base its
case for partisanship on reliable and well-founded claims to religious knowledge, such claims would be so inherently contentious that the expected
costs of basing policy on religious knowledge claims would always outweigh
the expected benefits" (Arneson 1990, 215). This fundamental idea of political tolerance in social policy is shared by Rawls: "Briefly, the idea is that
in a constitutional democracy the public conception of justice should be, so
far as possible, independent of controversial philosophical and religious
doctrines. Thus, to formulate such a conception, we apply the principle of
toleration to philosophy itself: The public conception of justice is to be political, not metaphysical" (1985, 223–51).

In many societies, this framework may not be appropriate. Before social
reform in Russia, the "common interests" of society were taken to trump the
interests of individuals in health care (as in other areas of social life). In such
a system, as Pavel Tichtchenko described it, "patients had no right to choose
physicians or medical institutions; informed consent was used only in cases
of surgery; patients or their surrogates did not participate in decision making
regarding the termination of treatment; and, the information in medical
files was closed to patients but open for state authorities" (1995, 75).

This lack of respect for patient autonomy will seem offensive to many in
the West, but it does not reflect malevolent intentions or an uncaring attitude toward a population. Rather, it reflects a differing political perspective,
based on collective good rather than individual good. Thus, individuals had
an obligation to undergo an annual preventive medical exam. Likewise,
concern with collective good over individual rights was evident in that individuals were not recognized to have a right to refuse an autopsy or organ
donation (see Tichtchenko 1995).

Some social systems that are closer to U.S. political ideology also emphasize a more collective perspective than than does the liberalism present in
American political institutions (see Hoshino 1995, 71–74). States Michael

Fetters: "In the past century, Japanese society has strongly emphasized the rights of groups and of society over the rights of the individual (though there is certainly a growing sense of individualism, especially in metropolitan areas)" (1998, 134–35). Although Japanese social and cultural systems are becoming more liberal, the historical approach of Japanese culture remains evident. Japanese culture has a long history of social and political structures based on a model of family authority, predating the restoration of the Meiji emperor by at least four hundred years. According to Fetters, "Until World War II, the Japanese constitution and civil code gave the legal head of the household virtual autocratic and absolute authority over persons who were quartered with him, and even over members of the legal household unit who lived elsewhere" (135).

Fetters goes on to observe that "respect for family authority, and the use of family relationships as models for other relationships in society, contrasts with models created in the US under the influence of the pioneer spirit and individualism" (134). It should not be surprising, then, that rather than a political and social framework emphasizing individual autonomy, Japanese culture operates within a model of family autonomy in which the family is deemed the locus of decision-making authority, for both competent and incompetent patients (132).

The impact of Japanese cultural history is evident in the attitudes and beliefs of the Japanese people. According to Kazumasa Hoshino, the Japanese concept of *wa** explains why people raised in Japan tend to adjust to the general opinion or consensus formed within a group to which they belong or are closely related (1995, 72). Culturally, medical decision making is understood as a *family* process, and patients themselves will normally insist on consultation with family or defer to family decision making in the interests of family harmony (71–73). Japanese law is thus heavily weighted in support of the family over individual family members (73).

In contrast, both the cultural history and political institutions of the United States are decidedly focused on liberal individualism. The liberal political framework is vital, and nonnegotiable, as a starting point in our dis-

---

* Hoshino explains that there is no precise English equivalent for this word. He uses the concept of "harmonious relationships" to approximate its meaning, which expresses a combination of conciliation, concord, unity, harmony, submission, and reconciliation.

cussion of bioethics decision making in the United States. Be we liberals, communitarians, communists, or other in ideology, we find ourselves in a liberal constitutional society. This context governs our social relations. Health care, as a social practice, is bounded by the fundamental political context within which it exists. In short, the role that moral beliefs play in bioethics will be limited, in a social context, by the political rights of individuals.

Imagine a health care professional who believes firmly that morality requires that we address overpopulation (often taken as a public health issue) and further believes that she is morally obliged by this requirement to address overpopulation through performing abortions on patients without their consent. Although her belief concerning overpopulation might lead *her* to seek an abortion, no matter how deeply she holds such moral convictions she may not impose those convictions on others in the manner described. So far as bioethics is concerned with the practice of medicine in a social (or clinical) context, bioethics must take seriously political boundaries.

Politically, we might think of the scope of bioethics as falling into three categories: (1) the prohibited; (2) the permissible; and (3) the required. The "prohibited" covers those actions, like seizing organs without consent, that are simply not allowed in a particular political society. The "required" are those behaviors that must be performed, such as treating (even uninsured) patients in a life-threatening emergency situation.* The "permissible" covers those behaviors that are neither prohibited nor required but are left to the judgment of the individual.

To be certain, the "permissible" is by far the largest category in a liberal political system. However, it is not all-encompassing. There are behaviors that clearly are prohibited or required, regardless of personal moral beliefs. The boundaries these prohibitions and requirements place on an individual's behavior and how these boundaries arise from a liberal concern to protect individual judgment are the focus of this book. Establishing these boundaries is significant in defining the scope of application of personal moral beliefs. It also results in conceptions of obligations and rights that protect individual judgment by reserving for the individual the role of framing decisions affecting her life according to values she adopts for herself.

---

*Such an obligation is mitigated by certain circumstances, as we will see in chapter 5.

Introduction

Liberalism and Rights

A fundamental feature of rights language is that every right represents a claim against others (Hohfeld 1964).* That is, if I have a right to something (X), possession of this right signifies a claim I have against others in regard to X. For example, a "right" to be free from discrimination on religious grounds provides me with a claim against others not to discriminate against me on the basis of my religion.

These claims against others result in rights-claims being attached to corresponding duties on the part of others. So, my claim against you for non-discrimination provides you with a duty not to discriminate against me. Because rights-claims attach to corresponding duties in this way, a liberal society has a special problem in protecting autonomy through rights: For every right-claim granted in the name of protecting one individual's autonomy, another individual's autonomy is limited through the corresponding duties. For example, my claim to nondiscrimination restricts you from acting in ways toward me that would constitute discrimination, regardless of your views concerning the justifiability, or desirability, of such discrimination.

Liberal societies often balance the rights-claims under which autonomy is protected by distinguishing between two types of "liberty": positive liberty and negative liberty. The most widely known and cited account of this distinction was offered by Isaiah Berlin in a paper entitled "Two Concepts of Liberty" (1969):

> Negative liberty: I am normally said to be free to the degree to which no man or body of men interferes with my activity. Political liberty in this sense is simply the area within which a man can act unobstructed by others. (122)

> Positive liberty: The "positive" sense of the word "liberty" derives from the wish on the part of the individual to be his own master. I wish my life and decisions to depend on myself, not on external forces of whatever kind. . . . I wish to be a subject, not an object; to be moved by reasons, by conscious purposes, which are my own, not by causes which affect me, as it were, from outside. (131)

* Although Hohfeld recognizes four uses of the term, what he calls a "claim right" is for him the "proper" use, with the others seen as "loose," leading to confusion of thought.

The negative notion of liberty emphasizes the lack of obstacles to doing what one wants. Freedom from discrimination in purchasing a house removes a potential obstacle to the purchase of a house and allows one to purchase a house, if one so desires, regardless of race, religion, or whatever characteristics are protected.

The positive notion of liberty emphasizes the presence of the resources necessary to do what one wants. Freedom to purchase a house in this sense implies that the financial resources required to purchase a house are made available. This distinction in what positive and negative liberty requires from others is important when we turn our focus to rights. Rights designed to protect positive liberty will place corresponding duties on others to provide the positive resources necessary to achieve our aims. Rights designed to protect negative liberty, however, will require only that others refrain from interfering with our pursuit of our aims.

When considering the distinction between negative and positive liberty, it is important for our purposes here to focus on the effect each form of liberty has on the behavior of others. At times, the negative notion of liberty has been understood in terms of being free from, and the positive notion of liberty in terms of being *free to*. As Joel Feinberg argued, however, these notions are typically two sides of the same coin: "The man outside a divorce court who tells us that he is now free (presumably from the woman who was his wife) has not communicated much to us until he specifies which desires he can satisfy now that he could not satisfy when he was married" (1980, 5). However we view the distinction between positive and negative liberty in terms of its affect on our *own* actions, it remains true that a negative notion of liberty can be distinguished from a positive one in terms of what is required of others for each notion of liberty to be realized. A negative notion of liberty requires only that others refrain from placing obstacles in our path; a positive notion of liberty requires that we be provided positive resources necessary to accomplish our aims. We discuss how health care professionals might have positive duties to promote our own abilities, and the degree of intrusiveness of each type of liberty on the aims of others, in detail in chapter 5.

Whether or not negative requirements are less intrusive on one's own aims, our society seems to take them to be so. The relevance of this feature for our political (especially legal) duties seems firmly to reflect the importance of the intrusiveness of political requirements on the aims of individuals for establishing the boundaries of such requirements. This general perception seems to be the approach recognized by the political (especially legal) structures in the United States, in which positive requirements are seen as more demanding on the aims of individuals, creating what Feinberg characterized as a perception that establishing a duty to aid is inconsistent with liberal social arrangements. This perception is so fundamental, that, as Feinberg states: "The common-law tradition has left unpunished even harmful omissions of an immoral kind—malicious failures to warn a blind man of an open manhole, to lift the head of a sleeping drunk out of a puddle of water, to throw a rope from a bridge to a drowning swimmer, to rescue or even report the discovery of a small child wandering lost in the wood, and so on" (1984, 127).

Positive liberty-rights are taken to require that others engage in activities that are motivated by the aims in question, activities thus reflecting the values embodied in those aims rather than the judgment of the individuals of whom the activities are required. Negative liberty-rights, on the other hand, require not the positive pursuit of any particular aim but only that one not interfere with another's pursuit of a particular aim. This is consistent with individuals adopting positive aims that reflect their own judgments. Although negative liberty-rights are restrictive in that one may not pursue the aim of thwarting the aims of others in protected spheres (those protected by negative liberty-rights), these rights do not require that one pursue a particular aim. You may still direct your life within the range of options available, given the boundaries of liberty-rights that protect others' ability to do the same.

In general, then, a positive requirement to act is one viewed by *society* as imposing the aim of the required act, unlike a prohibition, which does not specify an aim but only limits aims. That is, of course, unless the prohibition were so extensive as to leave available only minimal options; or the positive requirement so minimal as to hardly impose an aim at all.

For this reason, the rights designed to protect autonomy in a liberal society normally reflect the balance of liberties provided by negative liberty-rights (though not always; again, the degree of intrusiveness, rather than the "positive" or "negative" nature of the corresponding duties, is the salient feature). Importantly, the claim I make here is a political claim, consistent with individuals holding moral views that they understand to require, morally, the provision to others of resources necessary for positive liberty. Indeed, most of us view our moral obligations as exceeding our political or legal obligations. At a political level, however, no such moral perspective is put forth. Rather, what is advanced is a political structure designed to balance the requirements of competing moral perspectives held by different individuals living together in society. The perspective advanced, then, is a political perspective: that of liberalism, which itself supports only that no one substantive perspective should be given a "privileged" position.

Conclusion

Respect for patient autonomy in a liberal society like ours (which recognizes negative requirements as generally less intrusive than positive) emphasizes the patient's right to refuse treatment, a right derived from the concern that one's life not be interfered with through the imposition of medical treatment. At a political level, there is no privileged perspective that might justify the imposition of treatment. At the same time, the liberal concern to balance autonomy-rights can be seen in the recognition of the health care provider's right of conscience. That is, while the patient retains the negative liberty-right to refuse medical treatment, this does not translate to a positive liberty-right to demand treatments or procedures that the health care provider finds objectionable.

It is important to note, however, that negative liberty-rights do restrict the range of cases and ways in which a right of conscience might be exercised: a provider may not exercise this right in order to override a patient's refusal and impose treatment. (A health care provider might exercise a right of conscience to refuse to perform a requested abortion procedure, but the provider may not exercise a right of conscience to object to a patient's refusal of an abortion procedure in order to impose this procedure on the patient.) The recognition of a right of conscience is required by the "negative" nature of the patient's claim, but it is limited to the patient's being free from the imposition of the provider's values; it does not provide the patient with a positive right to demand that a given procedure be performed.

I

PATIENT AUTONOMY

2

PATIENT AUTONOMY
AND INFORMED CONSENT

ANY DISCUSSION OF BIOETHICS in the context of a liberal constitutional political framework must begin with an examination of patient autonomy and informed consent. Health care touches on value questions that are taken to be among the most important and profound in a person's life. How these values should be understood and defined will significantly shape people's lives.

Few patients have a sophisticated understanding of their condition or of treatment options. Patients depend to a great extent on their health care providers' judgment. Diverse cultural, religious, and individual value systems also significantly influence how judgments are made, and these value systems often differ between patient and provider. Sorting out whose values inform which decisions is a vital starting point for moral discussions, but the political context is also important. Given that a liberal, constitutional political context places autonomy at the center of any decision-making process, it is not surprising that as the scope of health care has increased, concern to protect the rights of individuals to shape their lives in terms of values they have autonomously adopted has increased as well.

My examination of patient autonomy and informed consent has a twofold aim: first, to explore the role of the concepts of patient autonomy and informed consent in medical practice; and second, to discuss refinements of our current understanding of these concepts that will make their application more consistent with the liberal, constitutional framework of U.S. society. The bulk of the discussion in this chapter centers on the first of these aims, elucidating the central role that patient autonomy has come to play in contemporary health care. I argue for two primary refinements to this role: (1) adoption of a subjective standard of informed consent that, while far from perfect, is the only standard that can be justified in a liberal, constitutional context that seeks to take seriously the protection of an individual's unique value system; and (2) the use of therapeutic privilege as an exception to informed consent only in conjunction with a patient's waiver of informed consent.

The Case of Lydia

Understanding the role that patient autonomy and informed consent has come to play in contemporary health care requires that we appreciate the ways in which an individual's unique values can influence the evaluation of burdens imposed by, and benefits gained from, various treatment options. This example from an actual case history demonstrates this point:

> An elderly woman, Lydia, is recovering from a minor stroke and faces the need for surgery. With surgery, her chances of having another stroke would be dramatically reduced and her life expectancy significantly increased. However, she would suffer some "minor handicaps" as a result; the medical staff emphasize that these handicaps will be minimal. Although she would no longer be able to undertake more strenuous physical activities, like working in her garden, she would be able to walk, participate in the care of her grandchildren, and even to drive. But Lydia does not wish to undergo this procedure.

Health care professionals, as well as family members, want to override Lydia's refusal of elective surgery. Their sincere conviction is that Lydia's decision is a bad decision and that her life after surgery will be better than she expects. They point to the fact that the "minor" handicaps will restrict only strenuous physical activities and will not inhibit her ability to perform normal, everyday functions or to participate in the lives of her grandchildren.

For Lydia, however, the ability to work in her garden is the most important ability she has. Caring for her garden is the only activity she values at this point in her life. In fact, she tells us, she doesn't even like her grandchildren! (She considers them "brats.") In short, the supposed benefits offered are, to her, not so enticing, and the burdens imposed through handicaps that will make gardening impossible are great. Lydia's unique values lead to a much different evaluation of what constitutes a burden or a benefit.

Is Lydia's decision poor because she ought to value caring for her grandchildren more than gardening? Should the family's wishes, or those of the health care professionals, be weighed against Lydia's wishes in order to determine whether she should undergo surgery? Or should Lydia be allowed to evaluate for herself what benefits are consistent with her life and what abilities she values? In a society that recognizes no privileged perspective, by what values do we evaluate the fundamental merit of a patient's decision?

It is precisely when there is disagreement about the merit of a decision that the rights attached to patient autonomy become important. We do not need a right of refusal when others share our values and agree with our decisions. We can see in the case of Lydia that without respect for patient autonomy, medical treatment might actually decrease Lydia's quality of life, or the value of her life, as *she* understands it. Recognition of patient autonomy demands that we allow Lydia the right to adopt her own values and to use those values as she evaluates the desirability of surgery.

Liberal Autonomy and Informed Consent

Medicine has a long history of paternalism. Although court cases can be found in the more distant past that uphold liberal rights in the context of health care (see Faden and Beauchamp 1986, esp. chaps. 3 and 4), the most influential and explicit cases recognizing patient rights have been more recent. Most early court cases related to consent were narrowly focused on the idea of obtaining consent (see ibid., esp. chap. 4, 119–25), rather than, for example, on what information is disclosed to the patient. This should come as no surprise. The practical importance of value differences is directly related to the treatment options and alternatives available.

Before advances in medical knowledge and technology, concern with how the patient's values might differ from those of the health care provider were of less practical importance, and questions about rights in the medical setting were simply far less pressing. If one's alternatives are to receive the one treatment option available, and thus have a chance of recovery, or to not receive treatment and surely die, there will be far less room for subtle differences of value to influence the outcome of the decision (assuming most people wish to have a chance of recovery). When artificial organs, transplantation, certain sophisticated surgical procedures, and other contemporary medical treatments did not exist, neither did the potential conflicts of value they entailed.

Today, however, the vast array of available medical options can infringe on personal values in important ways. Certain religious values, such as those held by Jehovah's Witnesses, are inconsistent with, and threatened by, many advances in medical technology. Likewise, the development of alternative treatments offers options that may be less "effective" from a purely statistical perspective, but that are better when considered in the context of the patient's own values and preferences.

It is not surprising that the evolution of health care, and in particular the technological and scientific evolution of medicine in the recent past, has been accompanied by a rapidly increasing recognition of the importance of patient autonomy and informed consent. Health care now offers the possibility of varied outcomes. In one instance, it may provide alternative treatments that more closely match the values of a particular patient. In another, a patient's quality of life may actually be reduced by, for example, prolonging death without alleviating pain and suffering, or by compromising certain abilities that a patient deems important in order to improve those abilities that others *except* the patient value more (as in the case of Lydia). As the capabilities of medicine evolve, the role of a patient's particular values and beliefs become more significant.

From Consent to Disclosure

The rise in medical knowledge and technology, and the subsequent rise in relevance of a particular patient's values, has resulted in more explicit recognition of a patient's right to define her own interests. This recognition, in turn, has led to a shift away from society's concern only that consent be obtained, to a concern that patients be adequately informed about their condition, the risks associated with a recommended treatment, alternatives to the recommended course of action, and the consequences of refusing recommended treatment.

Inadequate disclosure can result in treatment decisions that not only are counter to a patient's values but also reflect a less-than-optimal outcome in the context of the patient's values.

An elderly man faces the need for prolonged ventilator support in order to survive. Informed of this, he requests that the ventilator be withheld and that he be allowed to die. Concerned about his decision, the staff ask for an ethics consultation in order to discuss the choice with the patient. In the course of discussion, the patient explains that the burdens of being on the ventilator indefinitely are not worth undergoing at this point in his life. When asked if he wishes to be allowed to die, he explains that although he does not want to die, he would rather die than have "a tube down my throat for a long time." At this point, the procedure called a tracheostomy is explained, and the patient replies that he was not aware that he could be "placed on a vent without having the tube down my throat." He is very agreeable to trying the tracheostomy.

The original decision of the elderly patient did not reflect adequate information. Ensuring that adequate information is provided on, for example, alternatives and risks, is imperative if a patient's values are to direct the evaluation of treatment options. Controversy remains, however, concerning the standard of disclosure that must be met in the informed-consent process. Three standards are commonly proposed to define this aspect of informed consent: the professional practice standard, the subjective standard, and the reasonable person standard. Although each of these raises serious ethical problems, only the subjective standard is consistent with liberal social values.

Traditionally, informed consent has operated under a professional practice standard, in which both the duty to disclose and the criteria of adequate disclosure reflect the "customary practices of a professional community" (Faden and Beauchamp 1986, 30). The professional practice standard remains the most commonly recognized standard of disclosure (31), but from a liberal perspective it is fraught with problems. Two related problems are most serious in this context. First, the professional practice standard looks to

17

the customary values of medical practitioners (as reflected in customary medical practice), rather than to the values of individual patients, to identify information relevant to the consent process. This focus fails to grant patient values their proper role in the decision-making process. Second, given that the reform of medical practice in a liberal context is fairly recent, relying on "customary" medical practice as the standard of disclosure might mean that professional customs inconsistent with liberal social values would be perpetuated.

A patient considers a recommended bronchoscopy to evaluate a pulmonary nodule. There is no reason to believe it is an emergency, as the nodule is smooth and homogeneously calcified. Nonetheless, the procedure has been proposed for the following day. In discussing this option and obtaining informed consent, the physician goes over the risks of infection, the risks if a lung is punctured, and bleeding (in case of biopsy). She does not, however, raise the very slight risk of damage to the vocal cords, which could lead to hoarseness (in all probability temporary), as this risk is so small and "insignificant" that she feels it does not warrant discussion. Her colleagues also do not routinely discuss this risk, as they share her view that it is insignificant. Unknown to the physician, however, the patient is a part-time singer with several performances scheduled in the near future. If informed of this risk, the patient will likely wish to postpone the procedure until after these performances.

As we can see from this example, customary medical practice reflects the medical profession's customary views about what risks are significant. It also reflects the profession's views of what alternatives might be desirable and, ultimately, of what is in the best interests of the patient (as defined by "customary practice"). In this, the professional practice standard fails to account adequately for the patient's unique values and for how treatment will affect the unique life the patient has authored. The professional practice standard of disclosure, then, is fundamentally inconsistent with the concerns of a liberal society. By focusing on the customary values of those who practice medicine rather than on the values of individual patients, this standard threatens to undermine the liberal recognition of those very rights to patient autonomy that informed consent is designed to protect.

Furthermore, to the extent that customary practice ignores the values of the patient, reliance on this standard of disclosure will perpetuate nonliberal practices. In a profession with a long history of paternalism, this is not insignificant, as customary practice is likely to be heavily influenced by that history. The focus on the profession's values makes it likely that paternalistic practice will be perpetuated.

In contrast, the subjective standard of disclosure takes account of idiosyncratic values of the individual patient and requires that disclosure be based on what that patient believes is relevant to decision making. By shifting the focus of disclosure away from the customary judgment of medical professionals to the values held by individual patients, this standard also resolves the problem of perpetuating the customary values of medical professionals in the informed consent process. The subjective standard thus reflects, at a fundamental level, the liberal ideal of protecting an individual's right to author his or her own life.

The problem that arises with the subjective standard of disclosure concerns its practical viability. It is difficult, if not impossible, for health care professionals to know adequately the idiosyncratic values of every patient. A patient may have values relevant to a particular treatment decision of which the health care professional is entirely unaware. Especially in contemporary medical practice, physicians are expected to see many patients and scarcely have time to address adequately even statistically common fears and possible reservations while obtaining informed consent. It is unrealistic to expect health care professionals to do the "research" on every patient necessary to ensure that every idiosyncratic value is accounted for.

A third standard of disclosure seeks to address the problems of the previous two standards. The reasonable person standard requires disclosure of information that a *reasonable person* would take to be relevant to making a decision. Because this standard does not require the health care professional to uncover the idiosyncratic values of each individual patient—only that he or she be familiar with the concerns a reasonable person might have—this standard is viable in actual practice (though still more demanding than the professional practice standard). With its focus on the values of prospective (reasonable) patients rather than on the customary values of medical professionals, this standard avoids perpetuating nonliberal, paternalistic practices.

Nonetheless, shortcomings of the reasonable person standard make it inconsistent with a liberal social framework. The most important of these shortcomings is the vagueness of the concept of a "reasonable person." A liberal society lacks a privileged perspective on values by which we may judge a particular value system as "unreasonable." We might appeal to statistical commonality to define reasonableness, but again, a liberal society's concern to protect an individual's right to author his or her own life is not limited to statistically common lifestyles and values. A liberal society's concern is precisely that of protecting idiosyncratic values. The reasonable person standard will fail in this fundamental purpose.

All three potential standards of disclosure for informed consent contain problems, but the problems inherent in the professional practice and reasonable person standards are fundamentally inconsistent with a liberal social framework. We are left, then, with the subjective standard as the only standard consistent with a liberal framework. The practical viability of this standard, however, remains a concern.

To address the viability issue, we must look deeper into the liberal framework. In protecting the autonomy-rights of individuals, a liberal framework places on those individuals responsibility for authoring their own lives and behavior. The individual should not be seen as a passive receptor of information but as an active participant in decision making. Thus, it is consistent with the liberal framework to expect the patient to assume some responsibility in the informed consent process. I believe that the seeming impracticality of the subjective standard is, at least in part, due to a perception that the burden of accounting for idiosyncratic values falls entirely on the health care professional.

Informed consent is a process designed to foster communication between patient and health care professional, to ensure that health care treatment is, as much as possible, consistent with a patient's values and desires. In this light, the patient cannot be viewed as a passive receptor of information, but instead must be expected to participate actively in identifying fears and concerns related to health care treatment. For example, a Jehovah's Witness who faces a surgical procedure should be expected to help identify the relevant implications of her religious beliefs, or of any other idiosyncratic values, for health care treatment.

We cannot, however, assume the patient knows every potential relevancy of her values for health care treatment. The patient may simply be unaware, for example, that a treatment plan might involve the need for blood products. The physician must, therefore, make some effort to learn potentially relevant idiosyncrasies. This research is inevitable in a liberal society, where the protection of idiosyncratic values is of fundamental concern. The important point here, however, is that the process of accounting for idiosyncratic values is not a burden that falls solely on the health care professional. Treatment decision making is, in this real sense, a *partnership*, with both patient and health care professional assuming responsibility.

To be certain, the informed-consent process under the subjective standard of disclosure will not be perfect. Even with full participation of both patient and health care professional, there will be gaps in some cases in identifying how the patient's values are relevant to treatment decisions. The subjective standard of disclosure should be viewed as an ideal toward which to strive, with the realization that practical limitations will prevent perfect disclosure. Given the fundamental inconsistency of the professional practice and reasonable person standards with the liberal social framework, however, this flawed ideal is the best we have to protect the liberal autonomy rights of patients, even though full accounting of idiosyncratic values cannot be guaranteed.

Exceptions to Informed Consent

Five general bases are normally offered as potential exceptions to informed consent: threats to public health, medical emergency, therapeutic privilege, waiver of informed consent by the patient, and a patient's lack of competence to make decisions. In clinical practice, the most commonly invoked exception is the lack of competence, which I will examine in detail in the next chapter. Of the four other exceptions to informed consent, the most problematic in the context of the liberal framework is that of therapeutic privilege. As we will see, the inconsistencies of the practice of therapeutic privilege with a liberal context make this practice one that should be employed only in conjunction with a waiver of informed consent.

Overriding a Patient's Values: The Public Health Exception

A liberal society regards with suspicion any interventions that override the decisions of adult, competent individuals. Thus, restriction of an individual's pursuit of her vision of the good life is normally allowed only when her behavior might result in harm (or significant potential harm) to others. This "harm principle" was championed most famously by John Stuart Mill (1956), and more recently by Joel Feinberg (1984, 1985, 1986, 1988)* in offering an account of the criminal law in Millian terms.

In a Millian interpretation of the harm principle, the idea of harm relevant to justify interference is restricted to "other-regarding" behaviors. That is, interference, particularly coercive interference, is justified only when the behavior in question poses the risk of significant harm to others. Paternalistic intervention, designed to protect an individual from harm brought about by herself, is not legitimate.

Perhaps the clearest example of interference with an individual's autonomous decisions in order to protect others from harm involves public health intervention to avoid epidemics. Although a patient's right to refuse treatment is strongly recognized by society, this right is circumscribed when public health is threatened. In the face of epidemics, the state may interfere to enforce, for example, quarantine or compulsory vaccination. As recently as the early 1990s, an outbreak of tuberculosis in New York City resulted in the detention of individuals (Coker 2000). The justification of such action clearly lies in the threat posed to others in the community at large.

The harm principle, as a political principle designed to balance negative rights-claims, protects you from actions on the part of others which would impose the consequences of their actions on you. It is concerned, then, with the effects of one's autonomous decisions on the lives of others. Some have argued against this distinction between harm to self and harm to others. For Joseph Raz, "the only reason for coercively interfering with a person in order to prevent harm is that it is wrong to cause such harm" (1986, 415). This Razian reading of the harm principle focuses on the wrong that is avoided through the restriction of autonomy, rather than on the person toward whom this wrong is directed.

---

* This series of four books was published by Oxford University Press under the rubric "The Moral Limits of the Criminal Law."

Although Raz's approach to the harm principle might well justify overriding autonomy from a moral perspective (Agich and May 1997), its applicability to our *political* understanding of the harm principle will be far more limited. For Raz, the political notion of freedom rests on a perfectionist moral theory. His version of perfectionism relies on value pluralism, but for Raz this plurality of values is limited and objective, thus providing a privileged (albeit pluralistic) perspective. In this, Raz differs substantially from the sort of liberal political approach we are concerned with, which does not recognize a privileged position for any substantive view on values, even a view of pluralism.*

Reflected in the liberal harm principle is a political concern, understood in the context of the political balance of negative rights-claims in a liberal society. In this, it is not the moral wrong that results from a decision that is recognized through the harm principle. Rather, through the incompatibility of a decision or action with the political structure, one's claim to autonomy is balanced with the ability of others to exercise a similar claim.

The "harm" with which a liberal society is concerned must be understood as an imposition of values or judgment of values which inhibits, or even dictates, the direction of the lives of others. It cannot be a substantive, moral notion, because in a liberal society we cannot understand harm independent of an individual's judgment and aims. Harm must be defined in terms of the effect an action has on others' values, as defined by those other individuals.

Understood in this way, we can see why a decision to forgo treatment of a contagious, infectious disease could be overridden by other concerns. What is significant is not that a patient's evaluation that the burdens of treatment outweigh the consequences of the disease is deemed poor. Rather, the social effects of this decision impose on others the evaluation of burdens versus consequences and threatens harm to them.

The Medical Emergency Exception

The only exception to the liberal doctrine of noninterference in the absence of other-regarding harm is when the agent simply lacks knowledge

---

* This view has led to questions about the "liberal" nature of Raz's work. See Lomasky 1990.

that he or she would take to be relevant for deciding whether to engage in the activity in question. The best-known example of justified interference in Mill's work is the agent who is about to cross a bridge without knowing that the bridge is unsafe: "If either a public officer or anyone else saw a person attempting to cross a bridge which had been ascertained to be unsafe, and there were no time to warn him of the danger, they might justifiably seize him and turn him back without any real infringement of his liberty; for liberty consists in doing what one desires, and he does not desire to fall into the river" (1956, 117).

This exception to the harm principle is important for understanding the most common clinical exception to informed consent: emergency treatment. Mill's example contains two salient elements for justifying intervention. The first concerns the provision of information that is needed to adequately make decisions. This would be analogous to the duties of information required by informed consent, a duty that is itself grounded in the fact that an individual's judgment cannot be reflected in a decision if the person lacks an adequate understanding of the circumstances in which she "steers" her life.* (I take this up in much greater detail in the next chapter.)

Importantly, Mill's example involves more than the simple provision of information: in his example, Mill argues that it is justifiable to intervene or seize the individual in question to stop him from entering a dangerous circumstance. The reason such intervention is justified is the second salient element of Mill's exception: that action must be taken immediately if the danger is to be avoided ("[if] there were no time to warn him"). The medical emergency exception to informed consent is justified, in part, on similar grounds. Consider the conditions in which this medical emergency exception applies:

1. There is a clear, immediate, and serious threat to life and limb.
2. The time it would take to gain informed consent would seriously jeopardize the patient's hope of recovery.
3. The patient exhibits factors that may be undermining competence (shock, hypoxia, blood loss, etc.). (Wear 1998, 21)

Both the example given by Mill and the conditions of applicability of the medical emergency exception focus on the clear, immediate, and serious

* For a more detailed understanding of autonomy along these lines, see May 1998.

threat posed to the individual absent intervention and on the need to take immediate action to avoid this threat. Just as important to the justification of the medical emergency exception is the patient's inability to give consent (the third condition listed above). Here, it might be useful to anticipate a dilemma for health care decision making in a liberal framework, which I take up at length in the next chapter: decision making for those who cannot participate in their own health care treatment decisions.

Consider cases of forced treatment of certain populations, such as children or those with mental illness. In the case of children, the courts have limited, for example, the rights of parents who are Jehovah's Witnesses to refuse treatment deemed necessary to sustain their child's life. Likewise, our society allows for involuntary admission to a mental facility when an individual has the symptoms of a mental disorder to the extent that he poses a danger to others or, significantly, to himself. While at first blush these examples may seem counter to the liberal idea of noninterference unless harm is posed to *others,* the liberal political approach (respecting strong autonomy rights) presupposes that individuals are capable of directing their own lives (and of assuming responsibility for this). Children and mentally ill persons often fall outside this framework. We are forced to appeal to alternative frameworks for these populations. Important for our purposes here, however, is that it is not because society deems the Jehovah's Witness belief as wrong that we allow interference in the decision in question. Rather, it is because society recognizes that the affected individual does not fall within the parameters of the liberal political framework.

In times of medical emergency, we are often forced to resort to similar alternative decision frameworks. To require consent before treatment can go forward may well undermine respect for a patient's wishes. For example, faced with an unexpected heart attack, most people would want to be revived through CPR. But requiring consent in this situation, where obtaining consent is impossible, before CPR could be performed would be counter to what, in the absence of contrary information, we have every reason to believe the patient would want. Because we simply cannot operate within the parameters of the liberal framework when the patient is unable to participate in decision making, the most reasonable approach is to go forward with treatment until the patient *is* able to do so. Furthermore, this approach allows for a reversal of course, whereas allowing the patient to die would not.

These last points are important and should not be overlooked. That an exception to informed consent is justified in cases of medical emergency does *not* mean that informed consent continues to be irrelevant once the emergency has passed and the patient is able to participate in decision making. The following case is not uncommon in a clinical setting:

A nursing home patient has a cardiac arrest, is revived, and is admitted to intensive care. When she regains decisional capacity, she indicates that she wants aggressive treatment withdrawn. Physicians refuse, arguing that treatment has already been undertaken, and they cannot withdraw now.

Mill's example justified intervention only because we have strong reason to believe that, since the individual in question is unaware of the danger, that individual's actions are consistent with her wishes. Likewise, the medical emergency exception can be invoked only because we have reason to believe our intervention is most likely to be consistent with the patient's wishes. The individual in Mill's example, once aware of the danger, may choose to go forward anyway without further interference. Likewise, our nursing home patient, once stable and capable of participating in treatment decisions, should be allowed to reverse the course of treatment if that treatment is not consistent with her wishes and to regain authority over her own health care treatment decisions.

Exceptions Based on a Patient's Best Interests: Therapeutic Privilege and Waiver of Informed Consent

The exception of therapeutic privilege is based on the idea that a patient's "best interests" are served by withholding information from the patient. The reasons for this may vary, ranging from the fear that bad news will traumatize the patient to the fear that certain information will irrationally influence the patient and lead to bad decisions. The latter can be easily recognized as inconsistent with the liberal framework.

A model seeks treatment for a skin condition that poses minor problems in her career. The recommended treatment carries a slight risk of worsening the condition, but this risk is so slight that

---

the physician withholds this information for fear that it would make the patient anxious and might lead her to irrationally forgo treatment. Unfortunately, the very slight risk is realized in her case, and her career as a model is undermined.

In *Canterbury v. Spence*, the courts ruled that therapeutic privilege "does not accept the paternalistic notion that the physician may remain silent simply because divulgence might prompt the patient to forgo therapy the physician feels the patient really needs" (Faden and Beauchamp 1986, 38). As Faden and Beauchamp point out, if such an exception were allowed, it might "endanger autonomous choice altogether, as when the invocation of privilege is based on the belief that an autonomous patient, if informed, would refuse an indicated therapy for what the medical community views as incorrect or inappropriate reasons" (37).

The concern that information might traumatize the patient is more complicated. Here, it might be questioned whether information is being forced on a patient at a time or in a manner that the patient herself might recognize as contrary to her best interests. For example, in many Asian cultures, giving a patient bad news is thought to inhibit the patient's recovery or otherwise be counterproductive to the patient's well-being. It is thus standard practice to withhold bad news from the patient and to look to the patient's family for decision making. Because such cultural beliefs and practices often reflect the patient's way of life and values too, a liberal society should be sensitive to the possibility that the patient's own values dictate that bad news be withheld.

A Korean man is admitted to the hospital while having difficulty breathing. Diagnostic tests indicate he has lung cancer. The patient's family is insistent that he not be told of the diagnosis, and they explain their cultural practices in this regard. Physicians are worried, however, that the patient will be unable to make informed decisions without this information.

The patient was ultimately informed that diagnostic tests had been performed (which he already knew) and that results would be forthcoming. In a simple strategy to resolve the dilemma, the patient was asked his wishes concerning handling of the test results and about decision making for his health care. He was told there was a possibility that the tests could indicate bad news, and he was asked whether given his cultural beliefs, would he want to be informed about the results of the tests or should his family make decisions on his behalf. The patient confirmed the family's position that he should *not* be kept apprised of his condition (good or bad) and indicated that his family should make decisions for him ("I will just concentrate on getting better").

In cases like this, it is consistent with (indeed, required by) the liberal framework to withhold information from the patient. Importantly, however, the reason this is justified is not a straightforward one of therapeutic privilege. Rather, therapeutic privilege is itself justified by another basis for exception to informed consent: waiver of informed consent by the patient.

At first blush, the idea of a waiver of informed consent by a patient might seem inconsistent with the liberal framework. The responsibility for decisions that is assigned to individuals in a liberal society is not easily avoided. A deeper examination, however, shows that a waiver of informed consent can represent a decision strategy adopted by the patient, a strategy that reflects the patient's values and judgment and that the patient assumes responsibility for adopting.

Autonomous decisions reflect the agent's assessment of the "balance of reasons" for action (see May 1994), "reasons" here construed in the broadest possible sense. But in real life, an agent's determination of action does not always reflect a simple assessment of the balance of reasons (see Raz 1978; see also Elster 1979 and McClennen 1990). Consider that, we sometimes use indirect strategies or adopt "rules" that do not fit the model of a simple assessment of reasons. To account for these phenomena, Joseph Raz (1990) devised a model of "second-order reasoning," in which an agent forgos weighing the particular (first-order) reasons for and against a particular action, and instead decides through appeal to a (second-order) decision strategy.

Raz (1990, 39) explains second-order reasons as reasons either to act on particular reasons for action or to refrain from acting on particular reasons for action. Whereas a first-order reason affects our determination of action through the weight of that reason, second-order reasons affect our determination of action through the effect the (second-order) reason has on other (primarily first-order) reasons.* Thus, second-order reasons are formal strategies to be used to evaluate reasons in a particular way. They do not directly determine action themselves, but rather provide a formal mechanism for identifying *how* (first-order) reasons should be evaluated.

Raz gives several examples to illustrate the concept of second-order reasons. The first of these involves Ann, who attempts to determine whether to take on a proposed investment opportunity:

> Imagine the case of Ann, who is looking for a good way to invest her money. Late one evening a friend tells her of a possible investment. The snag is that she has to decide that same evening, for the offer to make the deal will be withdrawn at midnight. The proposed investment is a very complicated one, that much is clear to Ann. She is aware that it may be a very good investment, but there may be facts that may mean that it will not be a good bargain for her after all, and she is not certain whether it is better or worse than another proposition which was put to her a few days before and which she is still considering. All she requires is a couple of hours of thorough examination of the two propositions. All the relevant information is available in the mass of documents on her table. But Ann has had a long and strenuous day with more than the average amount of emotional upsets. She tells her friend that she cannot make a rational decision on the merits of the case since even were she to try and work out the consequences of accepting the offer she would not succeed; she is too tired and upset to trust her own judgment. He replies that she cannot avoid taking a decision. Refusing to consider the offer is tantamount to rejecting it. She admits that she rejects the offer but says that she is not doing it because she thinks the reasons against it override those in its favor but because she cannot trust her own judgment at this moment. (1990, 37)

The basis of Ann's decision to reject the proposed investment offer is not the weights of the various reasons for and against making the investment. Rather, Ann has a reason that affects the reasons for and against making the investment. That Ann is tired and cannot trust her own judgment is a second-order reason to not directly assess the balance of reasons for accepting or rejecting the proposed investment.

In Raz's example, the second-order reason functions as an indirect strategy. Ann obviously wishes to get the highest return on her investment. The determination of which investment opportunity will benefit her most would normally be calculated by evaluating each alternative in regard to the end

* I discuss the concept of second-order reasons in a medical context in May 1993.

to be achieved. However, because Ann is tired and does not trust her own judgment, she maintains that she will likely fail to determine correctly which investment would result in the best consequences. Therefore, she feels that she will benefit most by not attempting to calculate at this time which investment would be best for her, precisely because she does not trust her own judgment. This reason affects the weight of the reasons for taking or not taking the proposed investment by making them irrelevant to her determination of action.

Let us consider a similar example in medicine. In making health care decisions, many people might find that they wish to defer to the judgment of a physician, stating, in essence, "Do what you feel best, Doc. I trust your judgment." This represents an appeal to an indirect strategy, in which the patient feels her goals will best be achieved if she does not make health care decisions herself but rather defers to the physician. Perhaps she lacks an adequate knowledge of medicine or recognizes that because she is ill, she does not trust her own judgment. Therefore, she decides to defer to the physician's judgment and not to act on her own assessment of the reasons for and against various treatment alternatives.

The appeal to an indirect strategy is consistent with a liberal social framework, so long as the strategy in question reflects the individual's own judgment and values (see chap. 4 for a discussion of strategies that fail to meet this requirement). To the extent that a waiver of informed consent reflects the patient's judgment that she trusts the physician's evaluation of information better than her own, autonomy remains (as evidenced by the adoption of the decision strategy itself). Likewise, to the extent that therapeutic privilege is invoked as a reflection of the patient's own values (as it is in our case of the Korean man with lung cancer), it is consistent with the liberal framework. It is when exceptions are invoked that override the role of a competent patient that problems arise.

Conclusion

The rights granted to individuals in a liberal society—designed to protect an individual's ability to frame for herself those decisions affecting her own welfare—are most important when an individual's values and decisions differ from those of others. Since health care decisions are among the most profound in effect on our lives and welfare, the recognition of informed consent has become the most fundamental right of patients in the health care system of a liberal society. Informed consent requires that a patient be educated as to the nature, risks, and alternatives to a proposed treatment and be given the opportunity to decide for herself whether to accept or reject this proposed treatment.

The exact nature of the information disclosed in informed consent must be based upon a subjective standard of disclosure if it is to reflect the concerns of a liberal society (which are the basis of the informed-consent requirement). This standard, however, must be realistic in what it expects from health care professionals in their awareness of what a particular patient would take as relevant to decision making. Informed consent, then, should be a cooperative process—a partnership—between patient and health care provider. Likewise, exceptions to informed consent should be grounded in the same liberal concerns that underlie the recognition of the importance of informed consent. These concerns allow exception to informed consent when harm is posed to others, when a patient waives his informed-consent rights, and in cases of medical emergency. A final exception to informed consent—when a patient lacks the capacity to participate in decision making—represents circumstances that simply fall outside the liberal framework. It is to these circumstances that I turn next.

3

PATIENT RESPONSIBILITY
FOR DECISION MAKING

MANY OF THE MOST IMPORTANT advancements in providing humane and responsible health care in recent decades can be traced to an increased emphasis that has been placed on patient autonomy. As might be expected, the greater focus on informed consent has been accompanied by a set of problematic cases. We wish to recognize the autonomy of "competent" patients (and thus their corresponding rights), but we also have had to face cases in which allegedly "incompetent" patients seem unable or unwilling to make, or uninterested in making, "good" decisions on important issues with profound ramifications.

A 55-year-old man with advanced leukemia has undergone several rounds of chemotherapy. Despite treatment, the leukemia has not gone into remission. During this hospital stay, the man indicates that he will no longer agree to aggressive treatments, and he demands to be discharged home. Physicians are very optimistic about his prognosis with treatment, however, and are concerned that he is not making a "good" decision. Eventually, he is transferred to a psychiatric unit on an involuntary basis because of threats to "jump out of the window."

The patient's demands to be discharged home became more and more pronounced. A combined ethics-psychiatric consult was requested. Discussions with the patient disclosed that he felt "imprisoned" in the hospital. When asked about his threats to jump out of a window, he replied, "Yes, I told the doctor that I don't want to be imprisoned. I want to go home. If they don't discharge me, I'll jump out of a window and go home." Discussions also revealed an alert, oriented, lucid man, who had given much thought to his decision and had even prepared by "getting my things in order for my death" before this admission. He accurately volunteered the physician's prognosis should he not accept continued treatment. In all, the patient's decision seemed a reasoned decision that had taken into account all consequences of refusal. Nonetheless, physicians disagreed, continuing to point to an optimistic prognosis with treatment.

When others agree with a decision we make, we do not need to appeal to our right to make autonomous decisions. It is only when others disagree with us and we are unable to convince them of our decision that the right to autonomy is important. But it is precisely in these cases that we are most likely to be considered "incompetent." Because of this, the President's Commission for the Study of Ethical Problems in Medicine and Biomedical and Behavioral Research (1983) decided that judgments of competence should not be made on the basis of outcomes or content. Despite this, I will argue that the "standards for competency" offered in the biomedical ethics literature often "smuggle" concerns about the merit of a patient's decision into the idea of competency, preempting the patient's judgment by assessing that the patient lacks the capacity to make decisions because the patient's decision is not a "good" decision. This leaves patients in the precarious position of being deemed "incompetent" when their decisions do not conform to values reflected in these modified notions of competency and autonomy.

I argue that a standard of competency should not test the merit of a decision in this way. Indeed, absent a privileged point of view, it *cannot* do so. The concerns that motivate the weight we attach to autonomy require a test of *type* that identifies the patient as eligible to assume the kind of role we reserve for autonomy; but this, as we shall see, is much different from a test of *merit*. The distinction between testing the merit, or "quality," of a decision and testing the type of reasoning exhibited is quite important. Many standards of competency employed in the medical ethics literature inappropriately test "quality" in ways that, to various degrees, render patient self-determination meaningless.

In the medical ethics literature, a common strategy for dealing with patient decisions deemed "ill-advised" has been to refine our understanding of autonomy so that we might understand why certain decisions made by "incompetent" patients should not carry the weight prescribed by respect for patient autonomy. In this, the standards of competency have moved from the capacity to make one's own decisions and direct one's own life to the ability to make "good" decisions. That is, standards of competency are often used to assess the merit or quality of decisions made rather than the capacity of the agent to make autonomous decisions. Consider the following passage from James Drane: "A properly performed competency assessment should eliminate two types of error: preventing competent persons from deciding their own treatments; and failing to protect incompetent persons from the harmful effects of a bad decision" (1985, 17).

At first glance, this seems an agreeable statement. Surely we wish to protect *incompetent* patients from the "harmful effects of a bad decision." The problem arises when one then attempts to define competency apart from a traditional understanding of a capacity for autonomy. For example, Drane maintains that "the patient's well-being . . . also has to be considered in assessing competence" (1985, 18). In a later work, Drane explicitly maintains that the standards of competency he proposes incorporate a balancing of values rather than being a simple assessment of the capacity to make autonomous decisions, stating: "A balancing of values is the cornerstone of a good competency assessment" (1994, 157).

Drane is not alone in importing the notion of good decision making into the notion of competency. For example, Loren Roth, Paul Appelbaum, Alan Meisel, and Charles Lidz found that tests used by clinicians to determine competency include "reasonable outcome of choice," among others (Roth, Meisel, and Lidz 1977; Appelbaum and Roth 1981). Many of these tests assess not competency to make a judgment but rather the merit or quality of judgment. As Kenneth Kaplan observed, "It should be noted that assessing a patient's judgment is frequently referred to as testing 'competency.' Good judgment and competency are repeatedly used in the literature as synonyms" (1988, 202). Kaplan goes on to examine the judgments made by patients, but he cautions, "What is offered here is a method to test judgment. It is not a method to test competency per se" (203). The problem is not with an approach like Kaplan's, but with the failure of much medical ethics literature to distinguish these assessments properly.

Drane recognizes that different standards of competence are used in different decision-making situations, and he attempts to incorporate this into the discussion of competency. Drane (1985) offers a "sliding scale" model of competency, in which the standards of competency employed become more demanding when the consequences of the decision in question become more dangerous. His model seems to allow "autonomy" to pull significant weight when there is little risk, but when more danger is involved it allows health care professionals to require the patient to perform a more rigorous weighing and balancing, to demonstrate a higher level of understanding of treatment alternatives, and to better justify their decision.

Drane's proposed sliding scale involves three standards of competency. The first (which is the least stringent) requires minimal awareness of one's medical situation and simple assent. The second requires an understanding of one's medical situation and proposed treatment and a choice based on medical outcomes. The third (the most stringent) requires critical and reflective understanding of illness and treatment and a "rational decision" based on relevant implications, including *articulated* beliefs and values (1985, 19).

This sliding scale of competency seems to import a notion of merit through the seriousness of the consequences of the patient's decision. Drane's sliding scale would seem to vary the patient's competency to make decisions, even within the same case. Suppose I need to have a relatively safe procedure done, such as an appendectomy, in the absence of which I might face very serious consequences. Using Drane's scale, I could well be deemed competent to accept treatment (this would require only the least stringent standard), but incompetent to refuse treatment (this would require the most stringent standard). This should raise suspicion, for if one is eligible to assume the role of evaluating the treatment as desirable, one should also be eligible to evaluate the treatment as undesirable.

Not only does the sliding-scale approach give us this problematic manipulation of the ability to make autonomous decisions, it leaves us *still* needing a debate about when the consequences of a decision are serious enough to warrant employing a more rigorous standard of competency. What exactly does "more dangerous" mean? I doubt we would want it to consist entirely of the "likelihood of failure." The dire consequences of refusing the appendectomy, for example, include the effects of this decision on the patient's future health and quality of life and also an assessment of what is at risk, in both physical and psychological terms—an assessment of the "values" that are at issue. Any attempt, then, to invoke a sliding scale of competency will require a point of view from which to evaluate the seriousness of outcomes. Because establishing this point of view is reserved for the individual in a liberal society, politically, there is no *privileged* perspective by which to judge this objectively.

One approach to addressing this problem is to frame the assessment of outcomes in terms of "task competence." In a well-known work, Allen Buchanan and Dan Brock begin their discussion of competency by asserting that "competence is always competence *for some task*—competence *to do something*" (1989, 18). Buchanan and Brock develop a model of decision-relative competence from this, as "there is a substantial variation in the complexity of information that is relevant to a particular treatment decision and that must be consequently understood by the decision-maker" (19). Thus, different tasks will require different levels of understanding, so that competency can vary between cases, treatments, and circumstances. Like Drane, they develop a scale for competency assessments which varies according to the seriousness of the consequences. For example, you may decide that your 5-year-old child is competent to choose between a hamburger and a hot dog for lunch, but you would not think the child competent to make decisions about how to invest a large sum of money.

The term *competence* is often applied, in ordinary language, in the manner Buchanan and Brock describe: "Joe is a competent accountant." In this use, it is appropriate to maintain, as Buchanan and Brock do, that competence is task-relative. However, such a notion of competency is employed in a very different context from the idea of competence as the right to assume decision-making responsibility. Task-relative competence represents an assessment of an individual's skills—of the *merit* of Joe's work as an accountant. By contrast, in the context of the capacity for autonomy, competence is the eligibility to assume responsibility for decision-making that affects one's own welfare.

The distinction between these two uses provides a different interpretation to the limited competence that Buchanan and Brock attribute to children in the earlier example. Children are not politically eligible to assume responsibility for decision making. They do not, as children, possess autonomy rights in the way that adults do. Nonetheless, we often allow children to make decisions for themselves. When a child is allowed to choose between a hamburger and a hot dog for lunch, it is at the discretion and goodwill of the parents. Importantly, the parents retain the right to overrule the child's decision; the child, in being allowed this choice, is not considered to have become eligible for autonomy rights. Although we might employ the term *competence* to describe the child's ability to make this decision, it is not meant to denote eligibility to assume responsibility for one's life, and thus to ground autonomy rights. Other persons who are not eligible to assume responsibility are treated likewise. For example, state guardians will, in reaching a decision for a ward, look first to the ward's own preferences, so that these might be promoted to the extent possible (Turner and IGAC 1999). Though we often look to these persons' preferences when deciding for them, allowing them to express their preferences does not mean that we believe they are eligible to assume autonomy rights.

The importance of distinguishing the contexts for use of the term *competence* is related to the purposes the concept is intended to serve. To the extent that a "task" can be identified in the context of eligibility to assume responsibility for one's life and behavior, it is the task of providing the values that will frame one's life and serve as a foundation for determining behavior. The "task" for Buchanan and Brock is more specific: the task of health care decision making, relative to the particular health care decision at hand. Buchanan and Brock (1989, 21–22) take competence as directly justified by the values of well-being and self-determination (task-competence thus serving to denote the ability to promote these values). As one might expect, the values of well-being and self-determination may conflict in performing the task of health care decision making:

> As is well known, and as physicians are frequently quick to point out, the complexity of many health care treatment decisions—together with the stresses of illness with its attendant fear, anxiety, dependency, and regression, not to mention the physical effects of illness itself—means that a patient's ordinary decision making abilities are often significantly diminished. Thus, a patient's treatment choices may fail to serve his or her good or well-being, even as the patient conceives it. The same value of patient well-being that requires patients' participation in their own health care decision making sometimes also requires persons to be protected from the harmful consequences to them of their own choices. (30)

While ultimately I agree that well-being and self-determination are important, our concern for both competence and autonomy is tied to their importance as a presupposition for a *political policy* that assigns decision-making responsibility for matters affecting an individual's welfare. We adopt this policy not simply because we believe that recognizing autonomy will promote well-being, but because a liberal constitutional society reserves the role of decision making to individuals. In this, we make no judgment about the correctness or merit of the decision, even relative to the patient's own conception of her well-being. As Joel Feinberg (1986) noted, when a person's self-determination conflicts with his well-being, he has a *right* to choose in a manner we might think to be foolish. The political policy of recognizing the patient's autonomy reserves for the *patient* the judgment of how that patient's treatment will be determined.

While the "complexity of information" Buchanan and Brock describe may affect an individual's ability to make a "good" decision, it will not affect that individual's eligibility to assume responsibility for her life (the political policy that grounds our concern with autonomy). Consider that when a person "leaps into" a faulty investment without carefully considering her alternatives, we do not say her action is less than autonomous. We say it was ill-advised, but that it was *her* decision. Suppose also that her stockbroker advises some other investment. She may have as little understanding of the workings of the stock market as the "uneducated" patient has of medicine, may be as unqualified to understand the various principles by which the market operates or the jargon used to describe this as the "uneducated" patient is of medical alternatives or medical jargon. Yet, when her stockbroker advises her to make a certain investment or to reconsider buying a certain stock, she may act against the advice of her stockbroker even though she lacks an adequate understanding of the market, its jargon, its cycles, and so on. Indeed, she may act against the advice of her stockbroker even though bad financial decisions can be disastrous to one's life (it could be argued that bad financial decisions can be as disastrous as bad health care decisions; certainly, individuals have been known to commit suicide because of financial disaster).

We recognize that autonomous individuals may well steer their lives by immediate concerns, or live a "spontaneous" life, or make ill-advised decisions. We may take care to be sure that such persons understand that acting in this way is quite risky and may have serious consequences. But if they persist despite warnings, they retain the right to do so. When we choose to restrict the acceptable outcomes of a decision to "good," we restrict autonomy.

Autonomy involves steering the direction of one's life, determining how to behave, and deciding what projects to engage in. Elsewhere I have referred to this as being "helmsman" of one's own life and behavior (May 1994). Often, people *do* direct their life through rational deliberations, investigating and weighing various alternatives, and so forth. Indeed, we hold such decisions as the "ideal" way to guide our lives. But at the same time, in many areas (unfortunately, probably in most areas of life), the direction of our behavior does not live up to such ideal standards. When these situations arise, we *should* be concerned that a person understands the seriousness of her decision. And we *should* take care to warn her of what we see as the negative consequences. But allowing the seriousness of the consequences to prompt this concern is a much different matter from allowing the consequences to partially *define* competence. Our concern to warn against negative consequences should reflect, as it does for Mill, our desire that the person make decisions in the context of the world as it actually exists.*

Autonomy and "Sanity"

Where does this leave us in assessing the content of a patient's decision? Should *any* decision be taken as equally valid so far as its reflection of autonomy is concerned, just because the patient has expressed it?

Surely, certain limitations must be recognized for decisions that might be considered autonomous. However, these limitations concern the person's eligibility to assume responsibility for decision making in the role reserved for the individual by a liberal society, not her "qualifications" to make the decision in question "well." In this, competency will be concerned with the *type* of reasoning exhibited by the patient in question, not the *quality* of the decision made.

A liberal society is structured in such a way that the role of judgment is reserved for the individual. Again, because a liberal society lacks a "privileged" conception of the good on which judgments of what behavior should occur

* For a good discussion of "ignorance" of risks, autonomy, and responsibility in the Millian tradition, see Feinberg 1986, 159–62.

might be made, the role of providing the values on which these judgments are made falls to the individual. That is, because liberal societies lack a standard of the good by which "appropriate" behavior might be determined objectively, the individual must assume responsibility for the role of decision making. Responsibility, then, will revolve around the role of the individual's judgment in determining behavior.

Because autonomy is central to our understanding of ourselves and the ways in which we structure society,* we wish to take steps to preserve autonomy as a characteristic of persons. Indeed, the Bill of Rights attached to the U.S. Constitution is a tangible indication of the significance we attach to autonomy. To undercut this characteristic is to require a complete reconceptualization of how we identify values, account for why certain things happen, justify our relationships with others, and parcel responsibility. In this, we want to recognize the right to informed consent, and we are concerned to place limitations on servitude (e.g., we cannot sell ourselves into slavery), precisely because it removes individuals from the model of responsible individual judgment presupposed by a liberal society. The concept of responsibility attached to individual judgment is the foundational presupposition of a liberal society.

Competence, then, should serve as a condition to identify the eligibility to assume decision-making responsibility for value judgments: while it should not judge the ability to make "good" decisions, it *should* serve to identify the capacity for autonomy presupposed by a liberal framework. This is important, for the very social culture that presupposes autonomy, and thus attaches importance to its recognition, will set boundaries on the types of reasoning which are consistent with how we understand individuals within this social culture.

Consider an appeal to intuitions offered by John Martin Fischer. Fischer asks us to imagine that we discover that the behavior of a friend is being electronically manipulated by a team of scientists. These scientists have secretly implanted a device in our friend's brain which allows them to monitor the activities of his brain. Whenever our friend deliberates, the device is used to stimulate the brain to induce certain decisions. Fischer concludes that, on discovery of the deception, a fundamental change would take place in our attitude toward our friend's behavior: "At first it would be hard to know

* I have discussed this at length in May 1998.

how one would react to such an unusual situation. But, I think, once you had been convinced that direct manipulation exists, a striking thing would occur: many of your most basic attitudes toward your friend would change. Your friend would no longer seem to be an appropriate object of such attitudes as respect, gratitude, love, indignation, and resentment. Furthermore, it would somehow seem out of place to praise or blame your friend on the basis of his behavior" (1986, 9).

Fischer's example may seem to some to be far-fetched or a problem only in science fiction novels. However, variations of this change in attitude are apparent almost everywhere one looks. We do not hold insane persons responsible for crimes, as we believe them to lack control in some fundamental sense. We do not hold children responsible to the same extent that we do adults. We do not hold people responsible for behavior that is compelled, coerced, or performed out of necessity, all of which represent circumstances in which we recognize the individual's judgment as ineffective. As Thomas Nagel states, "It seems irrational to take or dispense credit or blame for matters over which a person has no control" (1979, 28).

Susan Wolf recognizes a similar requirement as a condition of self-control and responsibility (1987, 46–62). Wolf argues that while responsibility does not require *ultimate* control over one's "deepest self," it does require "sanity." She describes sanity as follows: "We may understand sanity, then, as the minimally sufficient ability cognitively and normatively to recognize and appreciate the world for what it is" (56).

The requirement of sanity is not a requirement that an agent's action merely be determined by her practical assessments. Rather, it is a requirement that these practical assessments be related to the world in an appropriate way: "Some insane people . . . may have complete control of their actions, and even complete control of their acting selves. The desire to be sane is thus not a desire for another form of control; it is rather a desire that one's self be connected to the world in a certain way" (Wolf 1987, 55). That "certain way" which constitutes sanity is through an "accurate conception of the world" (ibid.). This accurate conception involves the ability to recognize and appreciate certain fundamental values and actual states of the world.

In assessing this conception of the world, it is important that we appreciate the perspective from which an individual views the world, and how this will influence her conception.

An elderly Polish man is revived by paramedics and brought to the hospital after having a heart attack. As he recovers, discharge plans are discussed with his wife, who is also Polish. She adamantly refuses nursing home placement, and she demands that her husband be discharged home in her care. The staff are concerned, however, as they do not feel her decision is based on reasonable grounds, and they worry about her ability to make sure the patient receives medication regularly. They point to her claim that the paramedics "bit" her husband and to her explanation that her husband would not be comfortable in a nursing home, because "we know what doctors and nurses are capable of." They confirm that there is no evidence the patient was bitten and offer the woman's distrust of health care professionals as evidence of mental disorder.

To resolve the situation, an ethics consultation was called, and discussions were held with the patient's wife. It soon became obvious that she was not claiming that her husband had been "bitten" by paramedics, but had claimed that he had been "beaten," pronounced with a heavy Polish accent. In fact, her husband *had* been "beaten" by paramedics in their attempts to revive him. Still, concerns remained because of her somewhat odd interpretation of this act: paramedics were trying to revive her husband, not "beat" him. Further discussions, however, revealed a past that made this interpretation somewhat more reasonable and made clear her reasons for distrusting health care professionals: During World War II, she and her husband had been held in a Nazi concentration camp, where medical experiments were performed. This horrible experience led her to distrust health care professionals profoundly, and it explained her conviction that her husband would be very uncomfortable in an "institutional" health care setting. When this information was made available to the staff, concerns about her ability to care for her husband at home were alleviated, and the patient was discharged in her care.

The importance of this example is that it points to the ways in which a person's conception of the world may reasonably differ from another person's conception. This is important for our assessment of a person's eligibility to assume responsibility for health care decisions. For our purposes, we do not need to require an "accurate" conception of the world in some *objective*, metaphysical sense. Rather, we need only recognize that the very social culture that grounds the importance we attach to autonomy is one that understands the world within a certain framework. If we view autonomy as an individual steering the course of her life and behavior, then to act autonomously she must have a *reasonably* accurate conception of the conditions of the world that serve as the context within which she steers her life and behavior. To fail this is to be unable to serve in the role that society has reserved for autonomous judgments.

This notion of "sanity" is a technical notion that is concerned not with the absence of a psychological disorder but with the capacity to assume responsibility for the direction of one's life. It is important to recognize that this definition of sanity is consistent with allowing a person who has a psychological disorder to retain eligibility for decision-making responsibility. As well, some individuals who do not have a mental disorder will lack "sanity" because they do not adequately appreciate the world (e.g., children, severely mentally retarded persons, and patients who are disoriented). What is important is the person's appreciation of the world as it is presupposed in the context of the social and political structures that ground the importance we attach to autonomy.

It may be objected that the distinction I propose is bound to collapse, for one of the ways we commonly recognize insanity is through the content of decisions made. That is, the content of a decision is often indicative of whether a person has a "sane" conception of the world. This may be true in many cases, but it does not threaten the distinction I propose or diminish its relevance. What is important is not the content of the decision per se, nor the consequences of this decision, but rather that the content might indicate something else: namely, that the person in question does not possess a "sane" conception of the world. The quality or merit of the decision does not itself threaten competency; it only serves to indicate that something that does threaten competency might be present.

Is it possible to make a third-person evaluation of an individual's sanity in this sense, without using the merit of her decisions as the primary indicator? I argue that it is. That we make this kind of third-person evaluation of an agent's first-person assessments on a basis other than merit can be seen clearly in the example of criminal trials. A jury considers various descriptions of an agent's first-person intentions, assessments, and motives, and then decides which seems to best fit the case in question. In making these evaluations, there is an assumption that the types of reasons for people's actions can be understood, even though the particular motives in question often seem "bad" or even "foreign" to the jurors themselves. A juror can recognize that a sane human being may be moved to commit a crime by a particular motive, even though the decision-making procedure that results in this act may be viewed as very poor, ill-advised, or morally wrong. Indeed, the jurors may understand others as able to be moved by certain considerations for which they cannot conceive of themselves acting, without this being taken to indicate the individuals are insane. The competing descriptions of the defendant's motives offered by the prosecution and defense attest to the fact that a wide range of decision-making processes are consistent with the autonomous reasoning of the defendant. When an insanity defense is used, it is not argued that the defendant did not make a "quality" decision because, for example, she did not consider the alternatives or the consequences of her decision appropriately (otherwise, nearly all criminals would then be deemed "insane"!). Rather, the idea is that the agent lacked an appropriate conception of the world, a standard that allows for a wide variety of "bad" decisions being sane in this technical sense.

The jury example reflects that the standard of competence based on an assessment of the type of reasons and decisions acted on—and not on an assessment of the quality of the decision—is employed throughout the bulk of society. Consider an evaluation of a paranoid schizophrenic person. When this condition threatens responsibility, it is not because we look at her decision and deem her incompetent on the basis that her decision was not "advisable." Instead, our evaluation of incompetence is based on the idea of sanity as a reasonably accurate appreciation of the world as it is.

The assessment of sanity in our technical sense, then, is not based on the quality of the agent's decision or the seriousness of the consequences of the decision. A sane agent may well make decisions in a very poor manner. That she chooses not to carefully investigate alternatives, for example, does not indicate that she lacks a sane conception of the world. Likewise, if she possesses a "sane" conception of the world, she possesses this conception whether the consequences of her decision are considered "great" or "trivial." Assessments of sanity are an assessment of type, not merit. They require that the type of decision made reflect a capacity to steer behavior in the context of the world as it is understood by the social culture and political structures that reserve the role of decision making for the individual. Furthermore, these assessments of sanity do not require that the agent's steering reflect the "best" decision procedure, or even a "good" decision procedure. Indeed, judgment of the content of the decision and the procedure for reaching this is reserved to the individual. A person who decides to determine behavior through the advice of a friend and is then advised to engage in some crime will not escape responsibility for his behavior. So long as he possesses the capacity for autonomy, he may choose to determine behavior in this manner, but he remains responsible for his resulting behavior (just as a patient who waives informed consent in order to defer to a physician's judgment as an indirect strategy retains the responsibility for adopting this decision strategy).

As we have seen, autonomy is important for establishing *who* has responsibility for determining a person's behavior and the direction of that person's life. Because of the value that we attach to autonomy in our society, this responsibility carries with it certain rights and duties. In medical ethics, this responsibility is attached to such rights as the right to refuse treatment and the duty to assume credit or blame for the consequences of undergoing treatment for which consent is given. (Thus, informed consent has assumed a central role in discussions of malpractice.) In society generally, the responsibility autonomy engenders is attached to such rights as freedom of speech, the right to privacy, and the freedom to structure our lives according to values we choose for ourselves.*

Likewise, this responsibility is also attached to our eligibility to assume credit or blame for the consequences of our behavior. The law does not apply in the same way to children, insane persons, or people acting in overbearing circumstances as it does to most people: We do not hold children responsible to the extent we do adults; we do not hold people responsible for behavior that is compelled, coerced, or performed out of necessity. In medical ethics, we do not allow truly "incompetent" patients to assume responsibility for treatment decisions.

---

* For a good discussion of the role autonomy plays in grounding these rights, see Richards 1982.

Ultimately, however, the similarity between the conditions of *responsibility* in law and the conditions of *competency* in the medical ethics literature serves only to illustrate an important difference in the stringency of these standards of autonomy: the law requires nowhere near the stringent standard of competence employed in medical ethics. Imagine that the law required the same standard of understanding employed by sliding-scale standards of competency before a person were held "responsible." Ask yourself, how aware are you of the legality of various alternatives and the subtle ways in which apparently illegal activities might be legal through a more sophisticated understanding of the law? On the other end of the scale, are you sure that various behaviors you engage in everyday are technically legal? The popular phrase "ignorance of the law is no excuse" seems importantly relevant. To view people as responsible in law, we require that the appropriate information be available to them, and then assume that they are responsible for either making themselves aware of this information or choosing not to investigate. In medicine, if they choose not to investigate (i.e., do not properly "survey the alternatives" or "weigh the alternatives"), we often deem them "incompetent." This standard is certainly quite different. Few people have the level of understanding of their legal alternatives that is demanded of patients for informed consent by the standards of competency that are commonly applied.

Consider once again our reaction to bad financial decisions. We allow people who have a "sane" conception of the world to make bad, even disastrous, financial decisions. But we are reluctant to allow those who lack a proper conception of the world, such as insane persons or children (whose conception of the world is not fully developed), to assume full responsibility for such decisions. Clearly, what is at issue here is not the merit or seriousness of the decision but the ability of the agent in question to direct the course of her life, given the conception of the world that social structures presuppose.

A standard of competence grounded in an assessment of quality, merit, or seriousness of the decision misses the point of competence as it is understood in a broader social context. To be eligible to assume the role that is reserved for autonomous judgments in a liberal society, one must understand the world as it is presupposed in this context. Without this capacity, one's decisions simply cannot reflect a translation of one's values to the conduct of one's life. So long as an individual is eligible to assume decision-making responsibility, she may exercise the right to make her own decisions, whether her decisions are viewed as "good" or as "bad" by others.

The Incompetent Patient

Because respect for patient autonomy represents a policy for assigning decision-making responsibility, what becomes important is that notions such as competency assess the individual's eligibility for assuming this role rather than assess that "value," "moral worth," or "quality of life" will be promoted. The notion of patient autonomy denotes the right to make decisions for oneself, even if those decisions would be viewed by some as able to be made "better" by another. This is precisely why self-determination is most important when others disagree with our decision. To require that there be agreement for autonomy to promote an individual's well-being, for example, would trivialize the recognition of self-determination.

To this point, I have left unanswered the question of how we should approach decision making for patients who *are* incompetent (who do not possess the capacity to assume responsibility for steering their lives and behavior). This category of patients is not insignificant. It includes not only insane persons but also children as well as patients who are simply unresponsive or otherwise unable to participate in decision making.

Since a liberal society lacks a privileged conception of the good by which decisions might be made for these patients, how might we approach decisions for these persons and determine what treatments are and are not appropriate? The difficulty of this question is manifested daily in health care. Should blood products be denied to a child whose parents are Jehovah's Witnesses on the basis of the *parents'* refusal? Should a severely retarded individual be kept alive on a ventilator only to suffer the anguish of the final stages of cancer? Should an unresponsive patient be subjected to experimental procedures that offer increased hope of survival but with side effects that might make survival undesirable for that patient?

Because incompetent patients fall outside the liberal structure for decision making, other mechanisms must be employed to assume the role of providing the value framework by which decisions will be made. These mechanisms include social policies of parental responsibility for decision making for children (along with limitations on parental authority), guardianship for mentally impaired persons, and advance directives for end-of-life decision making. Each of these mechanisms is imperfect in fulfilling the role reserved for individuals in decision making, however, and so limits reflecting these imperfections are recognized.

For the most part, I believe these mechanisms represent good social policy for addressing these difficult cases Therefore, I will not attempt to offer prescriptive recommendations for addressing these cases in a liberal context (indeed, the cases fall outside this context). Instead, I interpret these mechanisms in terms of the concerns and limits of the liberal framework, and I offer some cautionary observations about the limits of these mechanisms. I concentrate here on guardianship, parental decision making for children, and surrogate decision making for health care in general, as advance directives reflect unique circumstances in representing articulated views of the individual who is now a patient.

The "Void" in Values Left by the Incompetent Patient

There is no "correct" mechanism for decision making for incompetent patients dictated by a liberal framework. Rather, these patients pose special problems precisely because they fall outside the liberal framework. We are left with a void in decision making when a patient cannot assume the role of providing the "values" that frame decision making, as there is no standard by which to evaluate options as appropriate or inappropriate.

As a practical matter, this void must be filled, for even a decision not to treat is a decision concerning the appropriateness of treatment. We must do the best we can to adopt policies most likely to advance whatever conception of the good that patient might hold. Before I turn to health care in particular, however, let us consider how decision making for "incompetent" persons is approached in society in general. In this context, guardianship and parental decision making for children are good examples.

Guardians may be appointed for a person (a "ward") who lacks decisional capacity for a variety of reasons (Turner and IGAC 1999). The individual may be severely retarded to the extent that he is unable to assume responsibility, may have a temporary condition that impedes his ability to participate in decisions, or may have health problems (such as Alzheimer disease) that undermine his mental capacities. When we are able to do so, we choose guardians for these individuals who are close to, or familiar with, them, as such persons are normally in the best position to know the individual's social history and circumstances, likes and dislikes, and what seems to constitute his "quality of life" (ibid.). If this kind of person is not available, a guardian appointed by the state will make decisions according to her best estimate of the patient's interests. This process normally begins with an attempt to identify and understand the ward's own values and wishes, to get a social history, and to ask the ward himself about his wishes (69). The idea that motivates these approaches to guardianship is that, even where a patient cannot assume a role of responsibility for his own life, the ideal of self-determination should be approximated as closely as possible.

As a general rule, we take most parents to be quite concerned with the interests of their children and we assume they are best positioned to know what these interests likely are (indeed, as parents, they might well shape their children's interests). A child's parents, then, seem a natural "guardian" to turn to when health care decisions must be made for the child (who is not eligible to assume the role reserved for individuals in decision making). This authority would be limited when, for example, abuse is suspected, or there is other evidence that the parent is not acting in the child's best interests. The important point is this: Although children are not "property" of their parents but independent individuals, they are not eligible to assume the autonomy rights that are granted to normal adults. The authority of parents over children is based on their role as the child's "guardian," granted in recognition of the parents' special relationship and concern for the child. This role is subject to social intervention.

Especially in circumstances that are irreversible (such as withholding or withdrawing treatment necessary to sustain life), it is likely that society will intervene and the courts will become involved. When decisions concerning withholding or withdrawing life support for a child are proposed, the courts will likely consider the child's maturity and the degree of development of the child's own value system in determining authority to make these decisions.

When we introduce limits on parental authority to make decisions for children (or on a guardian's decision-making authority), values are imposed on the decision-making process by society. This occurs, however, in the context of a void in the decision-making process, a void that we seek to fill through the best-available mechanisms, but a void that is filled imperfectly whenever individuals are unable to assume the role of decision making for themselves. The limitations we place on these mechanisms reflect our recognition that although these mechanisms are imperfect, they are most likely to impose values consistent with the patient's interests when these interests cannot be defined by the individual's own judgment.

Similar concerns influence our approach to surrogate decision making in health care. Two standards are commonly appealed to when a patient is unable to assume a role in decision making: the substituted judgment standard, which tries to identify the subjective values of the particular patient; and the best interests standard, which appeals to a more "objective" standard for determining what a patient might want. Of these, the substituted judgment standard is preferred, as the primary goal is to approximate the values and wishes of the patient when these can be identified. There are times, however, when we simply lack any knowledge of a patient's values or potential wishes. In these circumstances, the best interests standard is employed. In either standard, consistency with a patient's values is of primary concern.

A middle-aged man who is a chronic dialysis patient has a heart attack and is brought to the hospital. He falls into a coma and is placed on a ventilator. An hour later, the patient's wife appears and demands that all life support be withdrawn and that her husband be allowed to die. When health care professionals involved in the case hesitate, she produces a durable power of attorney for health care that names her as the patient's surrogate. The patient has expressed particular wishes in the document, however, which contradict the wife's demands. Both through agreement with "standard statements" and in his own handwriting, the patient has indicated that he wants to receive life support unless in an *irreversible* coma. Physicians explain that several hours are not enough time to determine that a coma is irreversible.

Here, information was sought from other parties, such as nurses familiar with the patient from regular dialysis. All information available indicated that the patient would wish to be removed from the ventilator *only* if the coma were irreversible. The wife was not allowed to withdraw the ventilator. Three days later, the patient came out of the coma. When he learned of his wife's demands, he immediately revoked the power of attorney.

This case is not the norm (far from it). Nonetheless, it illustrates the importance of recognizing that surrogate decision making is a "next best" option and should be approached conservatively. Normally, family members are particularly good surrogates. They best know the patient's unique values and lifestyles and are typically concerned to have the patient's wishes respected, even at the expense of their own interests.

The family of a dying veteran in a permanent coma requests that ventilator support be withdrawn to respect the patient's wishes. But they ask that the patient be transferred to a VA hospital first, as he had repeatedly expressed a wish to die in that setting. Despite the costs involved, and the fact that logistical considerations surrounding the transfer to a VA hospital would likely preclude the family from being present when the ventilator was withdrawn, they were not deterred from their efforts to see that the patient's wishes were realized.

Because families best know a patient's values, and in most cases are concerned to respect the patient's wishes, health care professionals normally appeal to the family as surrogate decision makers (just as parents are assumed to be the best decision makers for their children, even though there are some cases in which this is not true). Nonetheless, that surrogates are imperfect mechanisms to identify a patient's values results in limitations on their authority. In Illinois, for example, surrogates may make decisions to withhold or withdraw life support (absent an advance directive or explicit patient consent) *only* in certain defined circumstances. Under the Illinois Health Care Surrogate Act (1991), these circumstances represent a conservative approach, where life support can be withdrawn only when a patient has:

1. a terminal condition from which there is no reasonable prospect of cure or recovery, death is imminent, and the application of life-sustaining treatment would only prolong the dying process;
2. a permanent unconsciousness in which thought, sensation, purposeful action, social interaction, and awareness of self and environment are

absent, and which to a high degree of medical certainty will last permanently without improvement, and for which the initiation or continuing of life-sustaining treatment provides only minimal benefit;

3. an incurable or irreversible condition for which there is not a reasonable degree of cure or recovery, that will ultimately cause the patient's death even if life-sustaining treatment is initiated and continued, that imposes severe pain or otherwise imposes inhumane burden on the patient, and for which the initiation or the continuing of life-sustaining treatment provides only minimal benefit.

Two physicians are required to document that these conditions apply.

In some instances, we may lack access to family members who can identify a patient's values. We are then forced to appeal to a best interests standard for decision making. Because a liberal society lacks a privileged perspective through which to ascribe *moral* "reasonability," this standard normally appeals to statistical norms. This means that where clear norms exist (and a patient cannot exercise her right to choose contrary to the norm), we follow that norm, since the fact that it is a norm provides a (statistical) reason for believing that (absent information about the patient's specific preferences) this approach is most likely to reflect the patient's wishes.

Decisions under the best interests standard will "err on the side of life," because *most* people would, in most circumstances, choose life over death. Thus, we adopt policies, for example, that in emergency situations (where consent is unable to be obtained from the patient), the health care provider should first "stabilize" the patient and worry about potential idiosyncratic values later, when other standards or mechanisms might be applied.

Conclusion

Decision making for incompetent patients is especially problematic in a liberal social framework. Incompetent patients are unable to meet the foundational presuppositions of a liberal framework, and so fall outside the parameters of this framework. When a patient is unable to fill the role of decision making reserved for her in a liberal framework, we do the best we can to approximate the individual's interests as we believe she would define her interests. The mechanisms used to achieve this, however, are flawed, and so conservative limitations are placed on surrogate decision making.

Patient Responsibility for Decision Making

The concern to approach decisions concerning treatment in a manner most likely to be consistent with the patient's interests is reflected in the prominent role that advance directives have assumed. Advance directives take precedence over other mechanisms for decision making for incompetent patients. (For example, the Illinois Health Care Surrogate Act does not apply when a valid advance directive exists.) This is because advance directives are taken to be good predictors of what decision a patient would make were she able to make a decision. In this, they are the best mechanism we have for making decisions for patients who are unable to make decisions for themselves. They remain, however, imperfect mechanisms for filling the void left in decision making, and as such should be approached with some caution.

4

ADVANCE DIRECTIVES
Extending Autonomy for Patients

ALTHOUGH A COMPETENT PATIENT has the right to refuse treatment necessary to sustain life, for many end-of-life decisions we lack direct access to the
wishes of a competent patient. Some treatment decisions near the end of life
involve patients with severely diminished mental capacity (e.g., those with
Alzheimer disease), some involve patients who are unable to communicate
(e.g., some stroke victims), and some involve patients who are simply unable
or unwilling to participate in decision making owing to the nature or sever-
ity of their illness.

Most states now recognize the extension of a competent patient's right to
refuse treatment through advance directives, which allow a competent person to specify in advance an approach to treatment decision making for use
when she is unable to participate directly in the decision. This extension of
a patient's rights has been recognized at the federal level through the Patient
Self-determination Act (1990).

A question remains concerning how far this extension of the right to refuse
treatment should be recognized through advance directives. In particular,
how literally should the wishes expressed in an advance directive be taken?

An elderly woman named Claire is largely unresponsive and unable to swallow as the result of a stroke. Her overall prognosis,
though guarded, is reasonably good. Because she is unable to
swallow, she needs a feeding tube. However, Claire has an advance directive in which she indicates that she does not wish to
receive artificial life support, including mechanical ventilation

or artificial nutrition and hydration. This has been indicated by Claire's initialing a "standard statement" (one of three statements that indicate different "approaches to treatment" on the advance directive form). The patient's daughter insists that her mother did not wish to refuse nutrition and hydration. "I helped her fill this form out, and we discussed which statement to initial. We chose only this statement because, of the three options, it was the *closest* to her wishes. The statement does not reflect her wishes *exactly*. She doesn't want to be kept alive on a ventilator, but she *does* want to be fed—especially if she has a decent chance of recovery." Indeed, examination of the advance directive document shows three options for "approaches to treatment" which a patient might initial. These options are preworded standard statements, and no option exists that refuses mechanical ventilation but does not refuse nutrition and hydration.

The case of Claire illustrates a fundamental difference between the wishes expressed through an advance directive and wishes expressed by a competent patient. Because advance directives apply when a patient is unable to participate in decision making, in cases like that of Claire we are unable to ask for further clarification of the patient's wishes. For this reason, we should not recognize advance directives as equivalent to the decisions made by a competent patient. I believe there are good reasons to recognize advance directives in many (perhaps even most) circumstances, but I also believe there are good reasons to recognize the important differences between advance directives and the direct decisions of a competent patient, and through these to require that additional criteria be met before advance directives become operative in treatment decision making.

Many discussions of advance directives and self-determination focus on the question of personal identity (see Buchanan 1988; Buchanan and Brock 1989; Radden 1992): If the advance directive is to reflect patient autonomy, we must address the question of the identity of the person who issues the advance directive and her relation to the person who is to receive (or not receive) treatment through application of the advance directive. Although this is an important question, it is not the focus of this chapter. Rather, I consider whether, given the resolution of problems concerning personal identity, the advance directive *could* be considered to embody patient autonomy. Ultimately, I argue that it cannot. That is, even if the patient who is to receive treatment under the advance directive can be said to be the same person who issued the directive, because of certain defining characteristics of the application of advance directives, such application must be seen as "binding" the patient in a way that is incompatible with the patient's autonomy.

An advance directive might take several forms. The living will and durable power of attorney are the most common, but medical directives and values histories may also be forms of advance directives. Each represents, for the purposes of this discussion, a similar phenomenon: each is a commitment to a particular strategy for making health care treatment decisions when the patient is unable to make such decisions directly. The important issue, then, is whether an appeal to such a strategy represents the autonomy of the patient. The particular feature that makes an advance directive inconsistent with autonomy—namely, the inability to reconsider the commitment to this strategy at the time of application—is common to advance directives, regardless of the particular form of the advance directive.

Note that there are ways in which people may "bind" themselves which *are* consistent with autonomy. Thus, it is not *simply* the appeal to a strategy for making health care decisions which I find to threaten autonomy. As discussed earlier, commitments to certain types of strategies can be perfectly consistent with autonomy. Remember the example of the patient who, because she does not trust her own judgment, decides to forgo her own evaluation of particular reasons for action in this case, and instead to weigh reasons for and against treatment by appeal to the physician's judgment.

Importantly, however, the patient retains the ability to reconsider this appeal if she should come to lose confidence in the judgment of the physician or even come to decide that she does trust her own judgment. To remain consistent with an agent's autonomy, the strategy in question *must* include an ability to reassess one's commitment to the strategy, a characteristic that is absent (again, by definition) in the application of advance directives, of whatever form.

This has serious implications for the autonomous determination of action through various formal mechanisms and "strategies." Although all formal strategies reflect the agent's adoption of that strategy, the ways in which different strategies operate within the agent's practical reason can be very different. Some types of formal strategy for determining action are consistent with autonomy, while other are not. Because of certain defining characteristics, advance directives specify *how* the determination of treatment is reached (a formal strategy for determining action), but cannot reflect an *autonomous* determination of treatment. Put differently, because of the conditions that define the application of advance directives, they might be taken to reflect the agent's adoption of a formal strategy for determining action, but they do not reflect the *type of* formal strategy that would indicate the agent's autonomy in determining action itself. To understand this, we must examine how phenomena like advance directives fit into an agent's practical determinations.

Practical Reason and Strategies

Advance directives reflect a decision-making procedure to be used when a patient cannot make active decisions, allowing the patient to determine treatment through commitment to a particular strategy; that is, by reference to the advance directive (see Howell, Diamond, and Wikler 1982; Dresser 1984; Winston et al. 1982). As noted earlier, the concept of second-order reasons developed by Joseph Raz provides a model for understanding decision strategies as "second-order reasons," which replace an agent's evaluation of particular (first-order) reasons by allowing the decision strategy to identify salient reasons.

Although Raz's notion of second-order reasons is a significant contribution to philosophical work in the area of practical reason and action, there remains confusion as to exactly how we are to understand what a second-order reason is and how it relates to other reasons we might have for performing various actions. The examples used by Raz emphasize different aspects of the relationship of second-order reasons to other reasons for action but that diversity clouds the role of second-order reasons in practical reason. At times, it seems that second-order reasons are phenomena of indirect strategies to achieve an end that an individual may not achieve through direct strategy in determining action. At others, second-order reasons appear to impose obligations independent of other reasons and strategies for achieving a given end. In examining the concept of second-order reasons, I maintain that the apparent ambiguity in the examples of second-order reasons given by Raz stems from the different ways in which this type of reason might relate to other reasons for action. This distinction, which is not in Raz's work, can help identify when second-order reasoning reflects the substantive assessment of the agent and when it does not.

I examine two ways that advance directives can operate as second-order reasons within an agent's practical reason. The first, "indirect strategies," are consistent with an agent's autonomy. But the second, "relinquishments of judgment," are not. As will be shown, advance directives must be understood as the latter type of second-order reason, which is not consistent with autonomy.

A Second Concept of Second-Order Reasons

Recall that in Raz's example of the case of Ann (see chap. 2), Ann faced a choice between competing investments but did not trust her own judgment at the time a choice had to be made. She therefore adopted an indirect strategy to weigh (first-order) reasons for action. Raz has another example of a second-order reason, which seems to function in a slightly different way:

> Consider the case of Colin who promised his wife that in all decisions affecting the education of his son he will act only for his son's interests and disregard all other reasons. Suppose Colin has now to decide whether or not to send his son to a public school. Among the relevant reasons are the fact that if he does he will be unable to resign his job in order to write the book he so much wants to write, and the fact that given his prominent position in his community his decision will affect the decisions of quite a few other parents, including some who could ill afford the expense. However, he believes that because of his promise he should disregard such considerations altogether (unless, that is, they have indirect consequences affecting his son's welfare). Again, some will think that his promise is not binding, but that is beside the point. Our aim is simply to understand the reasoning of those who believe in such reasons, and it must be admitted that they are numerous. (1990, 39)

The agent's reason for action (Colin's promise) does not determine the agent's action directly but rather serves as a reason for the agent to act for a particular reason for action (that it is "in his son's interests") and excludes other reasons for action which the agent may have from his determination of action. Colin's promise influences his determination of action through its effect on other (first-order) reasons for action (it is a reason to act for a particular first-order reason and exclude others), and thus it is a second-order reason.

There are obviously many similarities between the case of Ann and the case of Colin. In neither case is the subject acting on "the balance of reasons," and in each case the second-order reason operates by affecting the weight of first-order reasons, making at least some irrelevant to the subject's determination of action. But there are also important differences. Foremost is that in Colin's case, the second-order reason in does not appear to function as an indirect strategy, but rather seems to change the normative situation by establishing new criteria by which to determine action.

In the case of Ann, the second-order reason did not change the end to be achieved (but only changed the strategy to achieve this end), whereas the case involving Colin is quite different. By placing an obligation on Colin to decide on the basis of his son's welfare, the second-order reason (Colin's promise to act only for his son's interests and to disregard other reasons) does not establish a strategy by which to achieve the end Colin sets, but instead *establishes* the end that Colin is to pursue.

These cases illustrate two fundamentally different ways that second-order reasons can function in an agent's practical reasoning. Indirect strategies do not eliminate an agent's practical evaluation from the determination of action in the manner that Colin's promise does. Although Colin's promise may be taken as a second-order reason because of his evaluation that it should be taken as such, it nevertheless then *replaces* his judgment in the practical evaluation of alternatives; the second-order reason identifies what is relevant to Colin's determination of action. This is similar in structure to voluntary slavery (and advance directives). Let us consider how.

The different ways that second-order reasons might function in the context of an agent's practical reason are especially important in understanding how "strategies" affect an agent's autonomy. Strategies that operate indirectly are affected by different sorts of considerations from strategies that operate as relinquishments of judgments (such as Colin's promise). A second-order reason functioning as an indirect strategy will be affected by indications that this indirect strategy is not the appropriate strategy for achieving the end desired. Thus, for Ann, considerations such as the unavailability of investment opportunities should she not choose one right away may indicate that a strategy of "not weighing the pros and cons for making an investment at the present time" is unlikely to give her the best results (either investment may be considered better than no investment).

Second-order reasons that function as indirect strategies may be undermined through reference to the end that the agent's own judgment establishes. Such indirect strategies allow the agent's own judgment to continue to determine action, as the application of the particular strategy in question reflects the agent's continued assessment that appeal to the strategy is the appropriate way to determine action. Because the second-order reason does not establish the actual end to be achieved, it does not inhibit the agent from changing her evaluation of various alternatives, including her evaluation of appealing to the strategy.

By contrast, those second-order reasons that function as relinquishments of judgment are not susceptible to such considerations. A second-order reason that functions in this way *establishes* the end to be achieved, preventing the agent's evaluation from influencing the determination of action. So although the agent's evaluation may establish the second-order reason, this kind of second-order reason establishes an end that is then independent of the influence of the agent's assessments. The *strategy* rather than the agent identifies to what to attach value. Although the second-order reason may be adopted on the basis of the agent's own judgment, the agent's judgment is then eliminated from the determination of action, (analogous to placing oneself on "automatic pilot").

Suppose Colin's promise to act on the basis of his son's interests is adopted as an indirect strategy. And in contrast to Raz's example, Colin does not hold a position of importance in the community. Because other influences on his decisions may be insignificant and because it takes a great deal of time to balance these considerations, Colin determines that in matters affecting his son, it would be best simply to adopt a strategy of acting on the basis of his son's interests. Since his son's interests hold great value for Colin, this strategy will most likely give the result Colin wishes (just as Ann's strategy was adopted because she believed it would most likely achieve her goal, given her tired condition).

Now suppose Colin's circumstances change, so that his position in the community becomes significant—so significant that the effect of his decisions on the community becomes, in the greater scheme of things, even more important to Colin than his son's interests. Colin will now likely determine that his strategy of always acting on the basis of his son's interests will not give him the appropriate result. That strategy, then, will probably be discarded.

If Colin's promise is adopted as a "relinquishment of judgment," he cannot discard the strategy on the basis of the change in his position in the community. His promise is to act on the basis of his son's interests and to take that as his end. His own evaluation of what is more important is no longer reflected by the strategy. The decisions made under the direction of this strategy are not *decisions* that reflect Colin's ends (although the adoption of the strategy itself does). Rather, they reflect the end established by *the strategy*. And this end might or might not coincide with Colin's. Evidence that it does not, unlike the effect of such evidence on indirect strategies, does not affect the strategy's application.

This type of strategy, in its effect as the agent's reasoning, is akin to voluntarily entering into slavery. The determination of behavior under slavery cannot be considered autonomous, even if the agent has voluntarily entered into this relationship. Although the agent may choose to have behavior determined through a slave relationship, the actual determination of behavior under this relationship is made by the master, not the slave. Importantly, the slave is obligated to act on the master's directives without the ability to reconsider this relationship; the behavior required need not reflect any ends of the slave. (Slavery here implies an inability to reassess whether to be in the relationship; a relationship that allowed such reassessment would not qualify as slavery. Even cases of slavery which are for a limited, specified time or for specified realms of life do not allow a choice to leave the relationship within the time specified or within the realm specified.) The slave may *hope* that the master's directives are such that they are consistent with the reasons for which she has entered into this relationship, but the obligation to do as the master directs is not contingent on this. Indeed, the obligation holds even if she finds the master's directives to be directly at odds with her reasons for entering into the relationship. This feature makes an appeal to this type of strategy inconsistent with autonomy.

Voluntary slavery might seem like an extreme example, but that only illustrates the serious dangers inherent in allowing the adoption of strategies from which a person cannot exit. We do not allow such extreme strategies in other areas of society. Some may consider marriage vows to be such strategies, but the legal availability of the option of divorce demonstrates that one cannot truly "bind" oneself into marriage without "exit rights." In medicine, the closest analogy to such a strategy would be requiring a patient to sign a "blanket consent" to treatment, regardless of any subsequent changes in circumstance or condition. Such an extreme "blanket consent" is simply not allowed in our society.

One may argue that the ability to relinquish judgment in certain areas of life is necessary to make life richer. If this is used as the basis for justifying advance directives, however, the concept itself should be removed from the realm of self-determination, with discussions of advance directives taken up regarding whether this is an area in which such an ability enriches life. To argue that an ability to relinquish judgment is an important aspect of a rich life is not to argue that relinquishing judgment is consistent with autonomy; rather, it is to argue that relinquishing autonomy is at times justified. There will remain many instances in which it is not justified. For some of these areas (in particular, for a phenomenon such as *true* voluntary *slavery*), I view this as unjustified precisely because it represents a relinquishing of autonomy and thus is inconsistent with the presuppositions of a liberal political framework.

Advance directives are not slave relationships. But as we have seen, the appeal to an advance directive represents a commitment to a strategy that is similar in structure to slave relationships, with regard to the strategy's effect on an agent's autonomy. One important difference between advance directives and slave relationships is that an advance directive may be changed at any time while the patient retains competency. However, at the time of an advance directive's application, the commitment to this strategy cannot be reconsidered. Thus, it is at this time the advance directive becomes analogous to a slave relationship. So long as the patient retains competency, for example, her active decisions take precedence over an advance directive. (I describe the important features of advance directives at the time of application in greater detail below.) Because this type of strategy cannot be reconsidered by the agent, in the manner in which simply deferring to a physician's judgment might be, the determination made under the application of the advance directive cannot be considered to reflect the patient's autonomy.

Commitment and Choice

In an interesting and thought-provoking article, Christopher Tollefsen (1998) criticized the model I offer here by giving several examples of how my critique of advance directives would also threaten other choices that most people would consider autonomous. I largely agree that Tollefsens's examples reflect autonomy. I disagree, however, that these are examples of the particular type of second-order decision strategy that I categorize advance directives as, and thus I do not believe that my critique of advance directives, if accepted, commits us to an unreasonably narrow conception of autonomy.

My view that advance directives fail to reflect autonomy is centered on the distinction I described earlier between two types of second-order reason: indirect strategies, which are consistent with autonomy, and relinquishments of judgment, which are not. At the heart of this distinction is the relationship between the second-order reason and the ends pursued by the strategy that the second-order reason represents: indirect strategies are means to an end that is set by and, importantly, continues to be advocated by the individual who adopts this strategy; relinquishments of judgment, once adopted, set ends to be pursued independent of the continuing judgment of the individual. The reason for this is tied to the individual's ability to reassess commitment to the decision strategy. This ability to reevaluate one's commitment to the second-order strategy is key for the strategy to be consistent with autonomy, and it is this ability that is lacking in voluntary slavery, due to the relinquishment of the ability to escape the relationship (if it is true voluntary slavery), and that is lacking in advance directives, due to the conditions of application.

Retaining the ability to reevaluate commitment to the second-order strategy does not threaten the "exclusionary" nature of second-order reasons or their ability to "silence," or simply reweigh, other reasons for action. The (first-order) reasons I may have for a particular action are a different set of reasons from those I have for adopting a specific strategy to weigh and balance these (first-order) reasons. Thus, one may retain the ability to reassess one's commitment to the second-order decision strategy and simultaneously exclude certain first-order reasons for a particular action through that strategy *while one is committed to it.*

Because autonomy, as I have argued, is reflected by an individual's assessment of the balance of reasons for action, the question becomes whether a decision reached through a second-order strategy reflects one's assessment of the balance of reasons for action (i.e., reflect one's judgment). We can divide this question into two parts: (1) whether the adoption of the strategy reflects the individual's judgment, and (2) whether the action determined under that strategy reflects the individual's judgment. I grant that all rationally adopted second-order decision strategies reflect part 1; the issue is whether the autonomous adoption of a decision strategy is sufficient to understand the action determined under that strategy as autonomous. I argue that it is not.

Let us examine Tollefsen's examples, to consider whether they represent counterexamples to to my model. Briefly, Tollefsen offers three types of considerations as examples of second-order reasons that reflect autonomy but that would not, he believes, be identified as autonomous in the model I offer. These include rational life plans (e.g., marriage; commitment to a profession), virtues (illustrated by the shaping of reasons for action), and law (which motivates compliance *because it* is the law). I examine Tollefsen's last example first, as I have taken this up previously (May 1997b), and the response to this example provides a basis for answering the others.

Tollefsen argues that the authority of law acts as a second-order decision strategy that would, in my model, threaten autonomy. This is because law, to be effective, must command compliance by virtue of the fact that something is required by law. The grounds for this requirement are most clear if we understand law as a system of coordination, ensuring compliance so that activities requiring coordination can be undertaken.

I agree that law is best understood as a coordination system and that, to serve its function, law must provide a reason to obey its directives *because* the law directs it. Consider traffic law. The good to be achieved through the existence of a body of traffic law is that there is a predictability to the driving behaviors of others (we all drive on an established side of the road). So, for example, if we turn a bend in the road, we can predict that should another car approach from the opposite direction, we would safely pass each other because we both know to travel on the right hand side of the road. Thus, we can safely travel from place to place, which we could not if there were no way to establish the "rules of the road." This good can be achieved only if I am confident that the rules of the road will be followed by others; this requires that others not constantly balance compliance against other reasons (such as the left side of the road might be more scenic).

Law, to be effective, must "silence" other reasons we may have for a particular action. It need not, however, silence the reason(s) we have for *adopting* the second-order decision strategy that law represents. Elsewhere, I have criticized Raz for extending the "exclusionary" nature of law beyond the first-order reasons for a particular action to the reasons one has for *adopting* a second-order decision strategy (in the form of law) that silences these first-order reasons (May 1997a; see also May 1998, esp. chaps. 5–7). Interestingly, for my purposes here, I argue that for Raz, this extension of the exclusionary nature of law has law claim the sort of all-encompassing authority that ultimately leads Raz to conclude that reason will not provide a basis for an obligation to obey the law. If we recognize the distinction I propose, however, we can understand law as a second-order decision strategy that *is* rational to adopt, *because* this distinction provides a way to understand the obligation to obey as not so broadly exclusionary. This is true, only if we understand law as the type of second-order decision strategy I characterize as an indirect strategy, rather than as a relinquishment of judgment.

This leads to Tollefsen's point: *Must* law, to the extent that it motivates compliance *because it is the law*, be characterized as the type of second-order strategy I deem "relinquishment of judgment"? My answer is no, and I have argued elsewhere (May 1997a) that understanding law as an indirect strategy better captures its exclusionary nature, if *any* limits are recognized, than does an understanding of law as a relinquishment of judgement.

Let us begin with the presumption that law *should* narrow one's range of choices by silencing (or excluding) certain reasons for action from our consideration, for the reasons outlined above. In my model, the reasons that law silences in this way are the *reasons for a particular action,* and it silences these *because* we have adopted a second-order decision strategy to obey the law (thus, because the law requires that we drive on the right side of the road, we "silence" our reasons to drive on the more scenic left side). However, law need not (and, I have argued, should not) silence consideration of the reason(s) we have for adopting this second-order decision strategy. If I adopt a second-order strategy of obedience to traffic law because it facilitates safe driving, I should be able to consider the strategy's failure to achieve this and reassess my commitment to the strategy on this basis (so, if traffic law actually makes driving more dangerous, I should be free to reevaluate the rationality of adopting compliance to its directives as a second-order decision strategy). This does not threaten law's ability to silence first-order reasons concerning, for example, which side of the road to drive on, so long as it is rational to adopt law as a decision strategy. Only if law fails, for example, to establish a consistent side of the road (and thus fails to do the things I adopt law for) is its ability to silence first-order reasons undermined. If I am not able to reevaluate commitment to a second-order decision strategy in this way, it is unclear how my own judgment might continue to play any role whatsoever (beyond the initial adoption of the strategy), and only through good fortune would the actions undertaken reflect any ends that I may set.

Perhaps the most important aspect here, and the reason I examined this area first, is that it illustrates how a second-order decision strategy—understood as an indirect strategy—will limit choice by excluding, or silencing, certain first-order reasons. This is important for addressing, at one level at least, Tollefsen's example of the virtuous agent. In the Aristotelian tradition, as Tollefsen correctly points out, a virtuous agent's perceptions of a situation will "silence" certain considerations that might otherwise have been applicable. Tollefsen takes this silencing to indicate that Aristotelian virtue is akin to advance directives or to voluntary slavery in my model. However, as we have seen above, second-order decision strategies need not be relinquishments of judgment to silence certain considerations. Just as one may view traffic law as an indirect strategy and nonetheless (through this) exclude scenery as a consideration that might inform a decision about which side of the road to drive on, one may exclude all manner of considerations on the basis of a second-order decision strategy adopted as an indirect strategy.

The deeper problem Tollefsen points to is that of the *shaping* of reasons by the very second-order decision strategies that silence them. This might indeed threaten to blur the distinction between indirect strategies and relinquishments of judgment for this particular type of virtuous agent, depending on the psychological processes involved and, even more important, on our understanding of the self. If this shaping dictates an individual's reasons without input from her own evaluative faculties, it would seem to replace the individual's judgment and thus be properly characterized as a relinquishment of judgment. I do not believe this process of virtuous reasoning threatens the distinction in question. I base this belief on a degree of agreement I have with Tollefsen's characterization of the self and with the Rawlsian "rational life plans" that are central to many person's lives.

Tollefsen argues that the conception of the self which underlies my position is that described by Michael Sandel as the Kantian conception: a self that is at all times independent of any choices it might make (1998, 410). By contrast, Tollefsen believes we should think of the self as something that develops over time and is constituted primarily through choices. Although I agree with the latter point, I do not agree with the former characterization of my positions. In fact, I have argued elsewhere that the Kantian conception of autonomy is inadequate on similar grounds (May 1994, 1998, esp. chap. 2).

The first premise of Tollefsen's argument is: "No self can pursue all possible ends, and no self can pursue any well unless it commits to those ends over other possible pursuits. To abandon one's chosen ends is thus in one way the reverse of self determination" (1998, 411). No one person can learn law, medicine, mechanical skills, and so forth, well enough to perform them all with an adequate degree of competence. Rather, we choose certain pursuits and appeal to the skills of others for areas we do not pursue ourselves. The circumstances in which one finds oneself will dictate that one appeal to various forms of authority and other decision-making procedures, and autonomy will be constituted not by a self independent of these circumstantial considerations but by a self that chooses the areas in which to develop abilities and the areas for which to appeal to authority and other procedures.

A self that develops over time, and through choices, will be partially shaped and changed (for future choices) by the present choices it makes. As we are forced to make commitments to certain pursuits that inhibit others, our range of choice options becomes partially reconstituted by the commitments. This relates intimately to Tollefsen's examples concerning Rawlsian life plans. Such plans call for interests to be ordered in a rational way, and through this to prioritize some interests over others in ways that will influence the future interests we develop (Rawls 1971). To illustrate this, Tollefsen observes: "In committing to my wife . . . I adopt a way of approaching future choice situations that eliminates, from the start, certain considerations that but for the commitment might have been reasonable for me" (1998, 409).

This example reflects a second-order decision procedure, as Tollefsen suggests. The question, however, is whether it represents an indirect strategy or a relinquishment of judgment. The key here is to ascertain whether the shaping of interests is done through the individual's development and reassessment, or through strategies *replacing* this development by establishing an end that then dictates the individual's interests. Consider the following passage from Tollefsen:

> In the effort at self-constitution . . . the scope of reasons that are salient for an agent will be increasingly diminished in some respects—as one commits to one's family, or one's profession, or the exercise of certain virtues, *those* will serve as second-order reasons exclusive of other possible reasons. And yet this reduced scope is precisely the consequence of self-determination. It is one's self as one has determined it that is now less interested in "self-interest" than in his commitment to wife and child, less interested in the allure of Saturday football than the *Nichomachean Ethics*. (1998, 411)

It seems incontestable that our commitments to second-order decision strategies affect our interests, desires, reasons, and ends, and that in doing so second-order strategies limit choice. It is not this effect, however, that threatens the autonomy of the individual who adopts this strategy, but rather the way in which the ends pursued by the strategy are set. A second-order strategy that is a relinquishment of judgment will do more than "shape" our interests and ends; it will *establish* these. In this, the ends we pursue are not subject to our judgments.

The issue becomes how we understand the shaping of interests, desires, reasons, and ends. Is this shaping dictated by the second-order decision strategy, or does it reflect a development, over time and through choice, of a self that is reconstituted by the prior choices it has made? It seems most plausible to me to understand this process as the latter. I may be shaped by a number of choices I make that are entirely unrelated to second-order decision strategies and commitments. Should I win the lottery, my range of options would increase drastically. Should I make a disastrous financial choice that bankrupts me, my choices would be drastically reduced and my "self" partially reconstituted. But neither of these need be dictated by a second-order strategy or commitment.

Current divorce rates demonstrate how few married persons consider their vows to be unavailable for reassessment, although even divorced couples have usually shaped their interests, desires, reasons, and ends significantly through the fact of marriage *while* married (and often beyond the divorce). Many people change careers several times. Our "life plans" seem subject to constant revision and reorientation, however slight or great these changes may be. These examples are evidence that the shaping of interests, desires, reasons, and ends by commitments of these types are not directed by the commitment, but reflect a reconstitution of the self in the face of changed circumstances one finds oneself in as the result of the prior choice to commit. Importantly, however, these commitments are subject to reassessment, and that they are at times dropped provides at least prima facie evidence that the commitments themselves are not dictating the judgment that reassesses the commitment.

Indeed, an inability to readjust one's life plan and commitments would seem odd, and such rigorous commitment to *any* strategy would seem at times irrational (Raz rejects a rational basis for an obligation to obey the law because he understands law as the type of second-order reason I call a relinquishment of judgment). If one believes that the self truly does develop over time, room should be reserved for the self to adjust, reconstitute, and reassess its commitments. This requires that autonomous commitments be subject to reassessment of the decision strategy adopted.

We have seen that advance directives, if they are to be subsumed under the right to informed consent and patient autonomy, should be understood as a strategy for determining action which amounts to a second-order reason. We have also seen that, although some second-order reasons function within an agent's practical reasoning in such a way that they are consistent with the agent's autonomy, other second-order reasons do not.

The characteristic feature of the type of second-order reason that is not consistent with autonomy is that, in replacing the agent's practical evaluations in the actual determination of action, the second-order reason identifies the "proper" way to determine action. In this, the agent's practical evaluations are no longer reflected in the determination of action when the second-order reason is applied. Rather than functioning as an indirect strategy that allows the agent's practical evaluations to "trump" the second-order reason, thus reflecting the agent's evaluation that the strategy in question is the proper way to evaluate what action to take, this type of second-order reason replaces further evaluations on the part of the agent from influencing the determination of action. Because the agent no longer continues to evaluate the strategy as the proper way to determine a given action, only the adoption of the strategy, and not the determination made on the basis of this strategy, can be considered to reflect the agent's autonomy.

Advance directives must be understood as the type of second-order reason that is *not* consistent with autonomy because the application of an advance directive is effective only when an evaluation on the part of the patient is impossible. For example, the Ohio State Bar Association and Ohio State Medical Association's "Standard Form for Durable Power of Attorney for Health Care" and "Living Will Declaration" forms explicitly state that "this power is effective only when your attending physician determines that you have lost the capacity to make informed health care decisions for yourself" (1991). Similar limitations are present in each state's advance directive forms. While it is true that you might regain the ability to make decisions for yourself, when you do, the advance directive is no longer effective. The defining feature of the advance directive's effectiveness is the patient's inability to make evaluations of her options, and this includes the inability to make evaluations that the strategy adopted continues to be the proper way to determine treatment.

Thus, a proper understanding of the various ways in which individuals might adopt strategies for making practical evaluations through the model of second-order reasons clearly illustrates that, while some types of strategy for making practical evaluations might reflect an agent's autonomy, advance directives cannot. This does not mean that advance directives should immediately be jettisoned from our concerns with "moral" health care. It simply means that advance directives, because of their defining characteristic features, cannot be subsumed directly under the right to patient autonomy. We must be cautious, then, in ascribing to advance directives the moral weight of a competent patient's decisions. The patient's inability to assess the application of the advance directive in a given instance places the patient in a situation with regard to the advance directive which is analogous to voluntary slavery. Advance directives do reflect the autonomous adoption of a particular strategy for determining treatment. But this strategy does not itself reflect the autonomous decision of a patient in identifying what treatment is preferred or consented to.

Advance Directives as Predictors

If advance directives do not reflect patient autonomy, why should they be given any weight? The answer to this question lies in understanding that autonomy is not a magical concept that alone confers value on informed consent. Autonomy confers value because it reflects certain cultural values and social structures. Advance directives might, in a different way, reflect these same cultural values and social structures, and thus warrant our attention.

It is not possible to incorporate autonomy into all systems or into some systems all the time. The medical system is one in which incorporating autonomy at times becomes problematic. For example, some patients are hospitalized because of psychological disorders that undermine their ability to make autonomous decisions. And, most important for our discussion, some patients are, due to a vegetative state, coma, or some other condition, unable to make autonomous decisions concerning continued treatment. Advance directives become important here.

As discussed, advance directives do not reflect autonomy per se, but they do offer a mechanism for incorporating what would likely be the patient's values and preferences in circumstances in which these values and preferences could not be incorporated directly. This provides a reason to give weight to advance directives even though they do not reflect autonomy per se.

Autonomy is important because a recognition of the unique values and beliefs of the patient is an immensely significant component of assessing the benefits and burdens of treatment options. Because the effect of treatment on a patient's quality of life will depend on the particular values that give meaning to that patient's life, we can be more confident that treatment offers appropriate benefits when treatment decisions reflect the patient's autonomous choice.

Given this, in cases in which autonomy cannot be incorporated, we need to closely approximate the autonomous choice the person in question would make, if a mechanism is available to determine what that person's autonomous choice would be. Advance directives provide precisely such a mechanism. By acting as predictors of what the patient would choose were she able to make a choice, advance directives provide a mechanism through which we can be more confident that treatment decisions will reflect an adequate assessment of the benefits and burdens of treatment on the patient's quality of life.

The reasons to recognize advance directives are indeed born of the desire to make health care decisions in a manner consistent with the autonomy of the patient, in circumstances in which autonomous decisions are impossible (as evident by the advance directive's applicability). The only alternative to honoring the advance directive seems to be imposition of a paternalistic decision by some third party (such as a physician or judge). Such an alternative would seem less likely to be consistent with the autonomy of the patient than honoring the advance directive. This argument in favor of recognizing advance directives is supported by a study published in the *New England Journal of Medicine* (Emanuel et al. 1991), which finds that advance directives promote the ability to identify a patient's preferences (either by providing a basis for predicting those preferences through the patient's prior articulation of preferences or by promoting discussion of those preferences with chosen surrogates).* In addition, this study finds that in the absence of an advance directive, third-party decision makers cannot adequately predict a patient's preferences on the basis of the patient's age, health, or other demographic features. Thus, the value of recognizing advance directives would seem consistent with the concern to incorporate patient self-determination into health care decisions.

It remains true, however, that advance directives do not reflect autonomy per se, but rather act as predictors of what autonomous decisions would be taken. This is most obviously apparent in the conditions of application for various forms of advance directives. Because advance directives are "next best" solution to decision making, we must be cautious in how extensively we recognize their application. The decisions reached through advance directives have profound ramifications, and protections are (and should) be

---

* In the absence of direct discussion with patients, substituted decision making is not likely to correspond with the patient's preferences. This may be relevant to the criteria we wish to impose on the recognition of a chosen surrogate's decisions.

built into their conditions of application which reflect our caution to "erring on the side of life" when patients cannot directly participate in decision making. This "caution" explains the different condition of application that different forms of advance directives have.

There are two primary forms of advance directives: the living will and the durable power of attorney for health care. A living will is perhaps the most widely known form of advance directive. It allows a person to specify in advance that she does not wish to receive health care treatment should she suffer from a terminal condition and death be imminent. Normally, the living will applies *only* when a patient is unable to make decisions for herself and suffers from a terminal condition in which death is imminent. A durable power of attorney for health care allows a person to specify in advance *who* should make health care treatment decisions for her if she should become unable to make these decisions for herself. Normally, the durable power of attorney for health care applies *any time* a patient is unable to make decisions for herself (thus, the patient need not suffer from a terminal condition and impending death). The durable power of attorney for health care provides the person named as "agent" with broad powers to provide consent or refusal for any type of medical care or treatment.

The reasons for the differences between the living will and the durable power of attorney for health care can be understood by reflecting on the role of advance directives as a next-best procedure for decision making when the patient cannot participate directly. Because the living will is an expression of preferences toward health care treatment made in advance of the circumstances in which it is applied, is does not provide for a way to assess unique circumstances that might affect a decision to accept or refuse treatment. Consider how one might respond to the abstract offer of a job, doing what one currently does but with a salary that doubled, or even tripled, one's current salary. In the abstract, and without knowledge of particular circumstances, many people would be inclined to say that they would accept such a job. But if more specific information is added, such as that the fact the job is located in a region where one does not wish to live or that would keep one away from one's family, one's attitude about the job's desirability might change.

The living will, by its nature, specifies health care treatment preferences in the abstract. Few people know the precise circumstances in which it might be applied, and so we are wary of "locking people in" to a decision made absent such vital information about the specific circumstances that might affect one's decision. Thus, applicability of the living will is limited to conditions where it is unlikely that changing circumstances would change the person's decision (terminal diagnosis where death is imminent). The durable power of attorney for health care, on the other hand, provides a way to account for specific information unique to a particular circumstance. Because the durable power of attorney for health care appoints an agent to make decisions for a patient, the agent can exercise an active judgment of the particular circumstances in reaching a decision concerning treatment. Therefore, the durable power of attorney for health care is far less restricted in terms of conditions of applicability.

The concern to protect against "locking a person in" to a decision made in advance of the circumstances can also be seen in the conditions required to revoke an advance directive. Although a person must be of sound mind to complete both the living will and the durable power of attorney for health care, the patient may revoke either document without being deemed "competent" to make decisions. Again, we recognize advance directives as a next-best solution, which states preferences in the abstract and in advance of the circumstances in which it will be applied. In this, advance directives are not informed by unexpected considerations or circumstances or by changes in attitude which might take place when a person is confronted with the actual experience of those circumstances. For this reason, we are careful not to commit to a decision with which people may no longer agree when the circumstances arise that make the advance directive applicable.

The Validity of Decisions Made under Advance Directives

The criteria used to evaluate the legitimacy of determining treatment by the mechanism in question differs between advance directives and active autonomous decisions. In the case of autonomous decisions, this criteria consists primarily of "competency to make decisions." Although the standard of competency is itself controversial, as we have seen, it is generally accepted that if a patient *is* competent to make a decision, her decision is the proper way to determine treatment.

For advance directives, however, additional criteria must be imposed, to ensure that the advance directive is a reasonable predictor of what decision the patient would make. We must recognize that the decision made in terms of the advance directive is a decision made before, and independent from, the actual conditions that obtain. Thus, whereas consistency with other decisions and prior experience with similar situations are not required for autonomous decisions to take precedence (unless inconsistency should call into question the patient's *competency*—but we shall assume here that the patient is competent), these factors may become important for assessing the legitimacy of advance directives as the proper mechanism for determining treatment.

Consistency with other decisions can indicate whether the patient had given sufficient thought to the advance directive to make it a reliable predictor of what decision she would make. It indicates that when similar values have competed, the decisions made are consistent with the decision expressed through the advance directive, and so the directive seems more likely to predict the actual decision that patient would make. Similarly, prior experience with similar situations indicates that the patient is aware of the factors that might "weigh in" in the circumstances, and so seems more likely to know what decision she would make.

In recognizing the validity of a chosen surrogate's decision (e.g., under a durable power of attorney), we should take care to see that the surrogate attempts to make a decision that is consistent with the patient's values and preferences. If the surrogate's decision is clearly contrary to what these values and preferences would likely be, we should question the validity of the surrogate's decision. For what reason is there to recognize a chosen surrogate's decision over a third party's decision if it is not that the chosen surrogate is, given that the patient chose her, most likely to represent the patient's wishes?

It may be objected that the choice of a surrogate decision maker may be based not on that surrogate's knowledge of the patient's preferences but rather on the patient's wishes that the decision reflect that party's values. A patient may designate a family member as surrogate because she wishes the treatment decisions to reflect her family's preferences. Such a basis for designating a surrogate is perfectly consistent with the model I offer, for it is quite appropriate for even active decisions to be based on a consideration of the preferences of one's family. If one's active decision would probably reflect the preferences of one's family, then to recognize the decision of a surrogate appointed for this reason is indeed to incorporate the likely decision the patient would make. What may become important is for a patient to identify *why* a particular surrogate has been designated, and then to examine the surrogate's decision in regard to its consistency with these reasons (in effect, establishing that the decision made by the surrogate likely reflects the ends for which the strategy embodied by the designation of this surrogate was adopted).

A full list of the criteria that should be required to ensure that advance directives are reliable predictors of autonomous decisions would require a discussion that incorporates studies by psychologists, health care professionals, health care clinicians, sociologists, and others. I will not attempt to offer a model of what is needed to establish the reliability of advance directives as such predictors. Rather, my discussion represents suggestions meant to provide an example of the types of criteria which might be imposed to recognize the validity of advance directives as the proper mechanism for determining treatment. The actual criteria imposed, again, must reflect empirical research into what is needed to establish the adequate reliability of advance directives to incorporate the patient's values and preferences. There is a significant lack of empirical research concerning these questions,* and therefore a need to redirect empirical research on advance directives toward questions such as, How should surrogates be selected to reflect the patient's values? How can advance directives be designed to reflect more stable preferences, those likely to still be held by the patient? What factors increase the likelihood that advance directives will be accurate predictors of the patient's decision?

Conclusion

Advance directives seem to provide a mechanism for incorporating the values of the patient into health care treatment decisions when these values are unable to be incorporated directly. This role establishes the value of recognizing advance directives and also establishes the need for additional

* See Lynn and Teno 1993 on this issue.

criteria to ensure the reliability of advance directives, because they do not reflect an autonomous decision concerning treatment per se. Recognizing this role can help us identify the types of criteria that might appropriately be imposed to recognize the validity of advance directives as the proper mechanism for determining treatment.

The implication of this understanding of advance directives is that there are a range of cases in which we might appropriately disregard an advance directive for reasons that would be inappropriate with respect to active decisions by the patient. This does not compromise the cultural values that ground our concern with patient self-determination. Advance directives are a mechanism by which we attempt to incorporate the values and preferences of patients in circumstances in which these values cannot be incorporated directly, and the criteria imposed reflect the appropriateness of advance directives for establishing what those values and preferences likely are. In this, disregarding advance directives because they do not meet the criteria meant to establish their reliability is no more a threat to the cultural values in question than requiring that active decisions be made by "competent" patients to be recognized as valid.

II

PROFESSIONAL RIGHTS
OF CONSCIENCE

5

BENEFICENCE, ABANDONMENT, AND THE DUTY TO TREAT

THE PRACTICE OF HEALTH CARE, with its long history of paternalism (in which the physician acted as sole arbiter in health care decisions), has only recently begun to recognize the important role of patient autonomy. Health care providers bring to the provider-patient relationship substantive moral beliefs of their own. These may be deeply held convictions, carefully considered, and well grounded. However, the "truth" of these convictions, as we have seen, is not recognized at a social level. Although these convictions may dictate the way in which that provider lives her life, and may also influence her understanding of her professional role (within limits dictated by the obligation to respect patient autonomy), they may not be imposed on the patient, regardless of how deeply they are held.

When the moral convictions of health care professionals come into conflict with a patient's convictions, it is often difficult to distinguish the obligations arising from one's substantive moral convictions from the obligations arising from a liberal political framework. A liberal society will require tolerance (mitigated by the harm principle), which is hard when deeply held substantive moral convictions are involved. Importantly, tolerance does not require that we accept, or agree with, the positions we tolerate; indeed, we don't truly "tolerate" that which we advocate.

Understanding the liberal obligation of tolerance requires that we recognize when a refusal to participate in a patient's treatment choice represents adherence to the professional's own right to frame her life, and when such refusal is an abandonment of the patient which constitutes intolerant denial of services. Helping health care providers distinguish among the obligations attached to their personal, substantive moral convictions, and the political obligations arising from a liberal social structure is one of the important roles of bioethics in protecting patients' autonomy.

To the extent that we attach importance to autonomy, we attach importance to an individual's ability to frame the values that shape her life by her own judgments. This protects both our right as health care providers to adopt certain values with which others may disagree and the patient's right to adopt values with which *we* may disagree. It is perfectly consistent to recognize a patient's ability to make decisions with which we might disagree, while retaining some discomfort with the decision precisely because we disagree. The rights attached to autonomy in liberal society require tolerance of alternative values. Again, we do not tolerate values with which we agree; rather, we tolerate values we do not ourselves share. Tolerating these values does not require that we accept them ourselves, but it does require that we recognize the rights of other to adopt them.

Recognition of a health care professional's conscience must balance the professional's autonomy-rights with obligations of tolerance in a liberal society (see chap. 6).But one must be clear about the nature of any positive obligations placed on health care professionals in a liberal society, for this defines the level of tolerance expected of a health care professional in a liberal political framework. For example, in the following case, is there a duty for the physician to continue to provide care to the patient?

Joe is a 48-year-old man who is experiencing liver problems as the result of heavy drinking. Dr. Smith has spoken to him on several occasions about the need to curtail his drinking and recommends that Joe join Alcoholics Anonymous and/or enter an alcohol rehabilitation program. Joe continues to drink and refuses to take steps to seek help. Dr. Smith, disgusted by Joe's abuse of his body and unwillingness to curtail his drinking, refuses to provide Joe with further medical care.

I will argue that there is a minimal "duty to aid" on the part of health care professionals, which in the clinical setting translates to a minimal duty to treat (absent mitigating circumstances, which I discuss below), through an obligation of nonabandonment. Our understanding of the duty to treat will be minimalistic; it should be seen not as an ethical ideal but rather as an examination of the professional's political duties — those derived from the liberal framework within which we have been working. One might, on the basis of one's own substantive moral convictions, regard oneself as having more extensive duties than those prescribed by the political framework (just as a person's moral duties as derived from her substantive moral views will likely be more extensive than the minimalistic "harm principle" reflected by political duties within a liberal framework). My primary concern is to examine the extent and limits of *enforceable* rights and duties in a liberal framework — the boundaries of personal moral views — consistent with the liberal aim of not imposing substantive moral perspectives and ideals of the good, either on the patient or on the healthcare professional.

Liberalism and the Duty to Aid

As we have seen, the negative rights granted to patients in a liberal society impose claims on health care professionals to respect patients' autonomy. The degree to which a positive duty to aid threatens liberal social arrangements is controversial. Many European countries have adopted legislation that punishes the failure to aid or rescue (bad Samaritan laws), but English-speaking countries have been reluctant to punish the failure to provide aid or rescue except where "special relationships" (such as a parent-child relationship) exist (Feinberg 1984, 126–86). As we saw in chapter 1, absent a special relationship, the common-law tradition does not punish even malicious failures to warn or rescue (Feinberg 1984, 127).

Feinberg notes that the reason for this reluctance to punish "bad Samaritans" is a fear that establishing a duty to aid is inconsistent with liberal social arrangements (although he goes on to argue for a "minimalist" duty to rescue). Such fear would not be surprising in a liberal framework, for the liberal framework allows no particular moral perspective, which might give rise to a positive requirement to aid, to be advanced. Heidi Malm, for example, believes that the difference between the stringency of the duty not to cause harm and the duty to prevent harm is because of the great value our society places on autonomy, and "it simply would not be fair to require persons to risk sacrificing their most important aims or interests in order to prevent a potential harm which they had no responsibility for initiating."*

The challenge that a duty to aid poses is twofold: (1) it must demonstrate the lack, or at least relative insignificance, of the imposition of value entailed by a duty to aid; and (2) it must demonstrate the positive requirement to aid through the harm principle or some other grounds that do not impose a conception of the good in a manner inconsistent with our liberal framework.

Minimal Aid and the Imposition of Value

Liberal societies are not seeking to eliminate completely intrusions on individual decision making, for even negative duties intrude to some degree on one's options. Rather, liberal societies seek to minimize intrusions through a balancing of interests in pursing one's aims, consistent with others not having aims or values imposed on them through a choice made by someone else (this balance, again, being reflected most notably in the harm principle).

Because liberal societies seek to minimize the imposition of aims or values (I use these terms interchangeably) on individuals, duties to aid are formulated in a manner that restricts such duties to the least intrusive, or to insignificantly intrusive, requirements (intrusiveness understood here as imposition of aims). Discussions of duties to aid in a liberal framework adopt conditions of applicability which reflect this.

Feinberg himself argues for a "minimalist" duty to aid (1984, 126–86), in which the costs of a duty to aid affect the applicability of the duty. As well, Patricia Smith (1990) defines the duty to rescue as a duty that holds in situations in which there is a clear and immediate need, where the agent is directly confronted with the situation (one is not required to search out such situations), where the situation involves the potential for serious harm, and in which minimal action is required for rescue (there is little or no cost to the rescuer). Compare this characterization to that of Smith's critic, John Whelan (1991):

1. There is sufficient reason for Jones to believe that she can prevent significant harm to Smith at little cost to herself.

* All quotes from Malm are made indirectly through Feinberg (1984, 167–68), who quotes an unpublished typescript, "Good Samaritan Laws and the Concept of Personal Sovereignty."

2. There is not sufficient reason for Jones to believe that anyone else will prevent harm if she does not prevent it.

3. The harm that Jones can prevent is not harm that Smith is morally required to undergo.

4. There is sufficient reason for Jones to believe that Smith would consent to having the harm prevented.

5. There is sufficient reason for Jones to believe that preventing the harm is in Smith's interests.

6. There is sufficient reason for Jones to believe that Smith cannot prevent the harm himself and cannot get anyone else to prevent it voluntarily.

For Whelan, these conditions are enough to impose a duty to aid if the cost to the rescuer is much smaller than the harm that she can prevent (454).

Although Smith and Whelan differ over whether the "costs" in question should be understood as relative or absolute, both understand a duty to aid as being restricted to situations in which the costs of rescue are small. This idea remains similar not only between these more recent philosophers but also to the characterization of a "Good Samaritan situation" offered by Wallace Rudolph more than thirty years ago:

1. The harm or loss is imminent and there is apparently no other practical alternative to avoid the threatened harm or loss except his own action;

2. Failure to act would result in substantial harm or damage to another person or his property and the effort, risk or cost of acting is disproportionately less than the harm or damage avoided;

3. The circumstances placing the person in a position to act are purely fortuitous. (1966, 242)

Generally, a Good Samaritan situation is one in which an agent is in a position to prevent harm to a (potential) victim with little or no cost to himself. The duty to aid in a liberal framework is thus restricted to circumstances of very little or no "cost." The idea of "cost" will be the focal point of such a duty. How we understand this concept will be key to establishing the consistency of positive duties with a liberal framework.

To be consistent with a liberal framework, the idea of costs that serve as the conditions of application of a positive duty to aid must be understood in terms of costs to a person's options, that is, how intrusive the requirement is in imposing aims on an individual. The reason for this is similar to the reason we must understand "harm" as the imposition of values: Because a liberal framework lacks a privileged substantive moral (or normative) standard by which evaluative judgments like "harm" or "cost" might be made objectively, any understanding of these concepts which might be employed in a liberal framework must be formulated in the context of the rights of individuals to provide the value framework(s) that affect their lives themselves.

This understanding of costs employed by a liberal framework to restrict the conditions of applicability of (potential) positive duties is itself a version of the harm principle. Rather than having an emphasis on restricting one's own actions to those that do not impose values (or "harm"; see chap. 2) on others, this version of the harm principle focuses on the imposition of values that one's duties to others impose on oneself. That is, one's political duties to others, formulated through a liberal society's balancing of the interests of individuals to structure their lives according to values they adopt for themselves, should not impose a conception of the good on that individual. Remember that the liberal emphasis on negative rights (which gives rise to the harm principle)—generally seen by a liberal society as less intrusive in imposing values on others (given that the rights-claims that one individual has are attached to corresponding duties on the part of others—is grounded in a similar concern.

The conditions of applicability of (potential) positive duties restricted to "insignificant or no cost," understood in the context of "costs" as the imposition of aims, reflect the same liberal concern to balance individuals' interests to structure their lives according to values they adopt for themselves which is reflected in the harm principle. The "insignificant or no cost" requirement restricts one's positive duties to others to times when the other's claims on an individual (arising from these duties) do not impose harm, or pose only insignificant harm, to the individual these claims are directed toward. Remember that the harm principle itself does not require an absolute absence of harm, only a realistic attitude concerning other-regarding and *primarily* self-regarding behavior. This attitude itself reflects a concern with *significance* of "harm".

Under these conditions, a minimal duty to aid might, in the abstract, be understood in a way that does not threaten to impose the pursuit of a particular conception of the good on health care professionals in a manner inconsistent with liberal social arrangements. This requires that such a duty be applicable only in circumstances of minimal cost (understood as the imposition of aims/values).

This still leaves us needing to demonstrate that a positive duty to provide aid exists, which poses a significant challenge, as our liberal framework presupposes no privileged moral perspective through which a failure to aid might be judged "wrong" (or an action as "morally required"). Such a positive duty offers special problems of justification not posed in recognizing negative duties. Heidi Malm offered these examples:

> Risk to my own health may justify my not donating the kidney you need to stay alive, but it would not justify my killing you if I needed your kidney in order to prevent the same risk to my own health. Or . . . suppose it would cost me one thousand dollars to alter my plans in order to avoid killing someone. This risk to my own interests would not, I think, relieve me of my duty not to cause a death. But if it would cost me the same amount in order to save a life (whose impending death is not my fault), then such risk to my own interests may be sufficient to relieve me of my legal duty to prevent a harm.

Establishing that positive duties might, under certain circumstances (of insignificant or no cost), be consistent with a liberal framework does not yet provide a grounds for recognizing such a duty. To this, then, I now turn.

Establishing a Positive Duty

A liberal framework does not attempt to eliminate the pursuit of social goods but rather restricts these pursuits to those consistent with the interests of individuals to structure their lives according to values they adopt for themselves. Within this context, it is often claimed that "social goods" either necessary or beneficial to the pursuit of *any* life plan that might be undertaken in a social context can be promoted, so long as these are consistent with an individual's political rights. John Rawls (1971), for example, argues that certain "basic" goods necessary to the pursuit of any conception of the good are legitimately promoted at a social level within a liberal framework.

We might say that a positive duty to aid provides a "social good" of rescue, for example, which when recognized only in circumstances of insignificant or no cost serves to enhance individuals' pursuit of life projects. Legal systems themselves are justified in the liberal context through the provision of security from violence, of stability of environment that allows one to formulate plans, and of conditions under which cooperative action might be undertaken; all of these enhance individuals' ability to lead autonomous lives (see May 1998, esp. chap. 7). Similar arguments might be made for the benefit of rescue where insignificant or no cost is imposed on the rescuer. This type of project might be pursued at a social level, if such pursuit is consistent with the political rights of individuals.

The next step in such an argument is to demonstrate that positive duties established on the basis outlined above do not themselves impose aims on individuals (and are consistent with a liberal framework). Feinberg has discussed extensively positive and negative (in his terminology, "affirmative" and "prohibitive") duties in terms of their intrusiveness on the aims of the individuals on whom these duties might fall. He argues that positive duties are not necessarily more intrusive than negative duties. As an example, he notes that certain "prohibitive" requirements, like the prohibition not to drive more than ten miles per hour in a school zone, significantly limit one's options. On the other hand, an "affirmative" duty for a bystander to warn a blind person that he is about to step into an open manhole "requires only a spoken word, which hardly limits his other options at all" (1984, 163). States Feinberg: "When one compares the degree of intrusiveness of a requirement to act . . . against that of a prohibitive restriction . . . one is as likely to find one as the other more restrictive of liberty, depending not on whether it is affirmative or prohibitive, but rather on its impact on one's options" (163–64).

I do not find this last statement entirely convincing; it hardly seems true that negative, or prohibitive, requirements are as likely to be found intrusive as positive, or affirmative, requirements, at least as far as this applies generally over a range of cases. Feinberg's examples seem to focus on particularly intrusive prohibitions and particularly nonintrusive affirmative requirements (though he does offer instances of particularly intrusive affirmative requirements), and it would require a much deeper study to establish such a claim. Nonetheless, Feinberg touches on an important point: It is not, ultimately, that a requirement is positive or negative that is important for its consistency with liberalism but rather the degree of intrusiveness the requirement imposes on the individual's pursuit of aims she has adopted for herself. Our primary concern is with the intrusiveness of a duty to aid in its imposition of aims on an individual. Feinberg's examples show that at least *some* positive requirements pose little imposition of this kind (e.g., the spoken word warning the blind person). Such positive requirements do not pose a threat to our liberal framework.

For those who find convincing the combination of the "social goods" argument and Feinberg's argument that "positive duties are no more intrusive than negative duties," the grounds for a minimal duty to aid consistent with a liberal framework is established. To argue for the consistency of positive duties with liberalism requires simply that we demonstrate the lack, or insignificance, of aims or values imposed by the adoption of these duties, along with the abstract benefits that rescue in these circumstances would provide to the pursuit of *any* life plan. So long as positive duties are consistent with the political rights of individuals, the social goods gained through a positive duty to aid might be pursued.

For those (like myself) who are not persuaded by the combination of these arguments the problem of establishing the grounds of positive duties in a liberal framework remains. Feinberg himself notes that our political and legal structures do not seem to accept his position, resulting in the reluctance to punish even failures to aid like the failure to throw a rope to a drowning swimmer. This is important, for I have attempted throughout this book to outline the boundaries placed on the social application of moral beliefs in society, which *in fact* serves as the context within which social relationships are governed. While this should not in itself deter us from recommending reform where social policy is clearly inconsistent with liberal requirements, it is also dangerous to rely too heavily on contested conceptual positions that are not themselves employed in the society in question. We should consider whether Feinberg's position is *necessary* to establish a positive duty to aid or whether a positive duty to aid might be recognized absent Feinberg's position, yet without enforcing a substantive moral perspective in a way inconsistent with a liberal framework.

One approach to answering this challenge might be simply to recognize that when one chooses to become a health care professional, one assumes certain responsibilities attached to that role which override what one would choose to do absent those responsibilities. This addresses our remaining obstacle to establishing a duty to aid by identifying the grounds for a positive obligation to aid by means of the health care professional's implicit agreement through voluntarily choosing to become a health care professional.

This approach, however, is fraught with problems. For one, it poses a dangerous slippery slope that threatens to dissolve a health care professional's right of conscience altogether. For if the patient's welfare is defined by the values that frame her life and that she adopts for herself, giving priority to the positive promotion of the patient's welfare over the health care provider's own negative liberty-rights obligates the provider to promote the conception of the good adopted by the patient and which constitutes that patient's welfare. This requires the health care provider to pursue conceptions of the good on behalf of the patient which the provider herself might consider morally repugnant (e.g., abortion or euthanasia). A waiver of this kind, which fails to recognize even the rights of conscience to refuse to pursue aims one finds morally repugnant, would almost certainly fail the "minimal cost" requirement, which plays a crucial role in keeping duties to treat consistent with liberal social systems.

Such waivers of negative liberty-rights generally are not allowed in liberal societies (we may not sell ourselves into slavery, even when "slavery" is the value one adopts for one's life). These general waivers pose a myriad of problems to a society structured in such a way that even fundamental concepts of responsibility presuppose that individuals assume the role of defining the value content of one's aims, a role that slavery, for example, preempts.* Consider the problems posed to society by persons acting under various "rigid" obligations, such as the soldiers at My Lai (see Taylor 1971) or judges ruling within a Nazi legal system (see Conot 1983). These situations pose great difficulty for our understanding of behavior, and particularly of responsibility for behavior, precisely because the autonomy that is so deeply embedded in our social culture, seems lacking. Such general waivers of judgment represent a much different type of waiver than a patient's decision to defer to a physician's judgment in waiving informed consent.

Recall that a waiver of informed consent represents an indirect decision strategy based upon the concept of second-order reasons. This type of reasoning is consistent with a liberal framework as long as the individual retains

* For a full discussion of the problems posed to liberal societies by these general "waivers" and why they are inconsistent with liberal social structures, see May 1998.

final authority in "exiting" from the strategy, thus retaining authority over when the strategy is employed in particular cases. I also identified another type of second-order decision strategy (akin to entering into a "slave contract," where one cannot determine whether the strategy is applied in particular cases) which is *not* consistent with a liberal framework. A general waiver of negative liberty-rights removes the individual from the decision process (one cannot determine if the strategy is applied in particular cases), and thus is inconsistent with a liberal framework.

While choosing to pursue a certain profession will surely place *some* obligations on professionals, it does not follow that it is permissible to require that someone who wishes to have a career in health care be willing to waive her negative liberty-rights to pursue a conception of the good which *she* adopts (consistent with not imposing this conception of the good on the patient). Our challenge is to see whether an understanding of a minimal duty to aid or treat might be consistent with the liberal framework we have adopted.

My approach is to examine the obligations that might arise from the nature of the physician-patient relationship. If this relationship constitutes a "special relationship," requiring certain positive duties (much as a parent-child relationship constitutes a "special relationship" requiring positive duties of the parent toward the child, neglect of which are punishable), we can analyze the nature of these duties in the context of this relationship. Ultimately, I argue that the physician-patient relationship does constitute a "special relationship" and that beneficence is a central feature of this relationship, resulting in a minimal duty to treat mitigated by a recognition of professional rights of conscience consistent with our liberal framework.

Abandonment and Beneficence

George Annas (1975, 1993)* has written extensively about the political and legal nature of the physician-patient relationship. He describes the general obligations arising from this relationship in society: "American common law supports the traditional proposition that, absent some special relationship, no citizen owes any other citizen anything. . . . As applied to

---

* The 1993 *Standard of Care* collects Annas's work from various publications over a number of years.

health care and medicine, the general rule, sometimes denoted the 'no duty rule,' is that a health care professional is not obligated to treat any particular patient in the absence of some prior agreement or specific legal requirement" (1993, 121). This would seem consistent with our worry that requiring health care professionals to waive their negative liberty-rights would be inconsistent with liberal society. Although there are exceptions to the rule requiring a duty to treat even absent a special relationship, these exceptions involve crisis situations and are generally restricted to special contexts, such as an emergency room (121–22). They do not even extend, in most states, to physicians who come across an emergency outside the clinical setting.* The idea behind the duty to treat in the emergency room is to recognize the special circumstance of emergency situations, in which the patient has no time or ability to find alternative care,† and the explicit recognition by providers in such a setting that these special circumstances are present (and limited).

There is no generally recognized duty for physicians to provide treatment in most circumstances. This changes drastically once a physician-patient relationship is formed. According to Annas, "A patient's right to treatment is greatly enhanced after the establishment of a relationship with a particular physician or hospital. This is because after a voluntary provider-patient relationship has been established, the provider has a duty not to abandon the patient" (1993, 122).

This obligation is quite apparent, for example, in Illinois law: "As a general rule, once the physician-patient relationship has been established, physicians are under an obligation to attend the patient as long as the patient's condition requires" (LeBlang, Basanta, and Kane 1996, 733). At first blush, this duty to treat may seem nothing more than the result of a contractual agreement. The relationship in question is often treated, for legal purposes, in contractual terms, but I argue that the duties in question reflect more the nature of the relationship than any explicit contract. For one thing, rarely does a specified contract exist between physician and patient. The formation of the relationship itself seems more the result of the recognized nature

---

* Five states have positive good Samaritan requirements: Vermont, Massachusetts, Minnesota, Rhode Island, and Wisconsin. See McIntyre 1994.

† There are exceptions even to the duty to treat in an emergency room setting when significant harm is posed to the professional. See Annas 1993, chap. 9.

of the practice of medicine than of any negotiated contractual arrangement. Consider the variety of ways in which a physician-patient relationship might be formed: "[A provider-patient] relationship is always formed when a physician agrees to examine or treat a patient for a specific ailment. This will usually involve a face-to-face meeting. But at least one case has held that a doctor-patient relationship can be formed simply by making an appointment with a patient for an office visit, at least where the appointment relates to a specific condition mentioned by the patient over the telephone seeking the appointment" (Annas 1993, 122). Illinois law is replete with examples in which a physician-patient relationship is recognized despite the absence of mutual consent (e.g., in the case of an unconscious patient, or in some cases for physicians examining a patient at the behest of a third party, such as an insurance company) (see LeBlang, Basanta, and Kane 1996, 677–82).

That the physician stands in a "special relationship" to the patient and this gives rise to some positive requirements is clear. But the exact nature of this relationship and the particular duties it gives rise to deserve more attention. Because health care providers can be said to stand in a special relationship with patients, I depart in one significant way from an important element of the duty to aid as it is understood in a broader social context (which supposes there is no special relationship between parties). This departure is important because beneficence is a key feature of this special relationship, providing a reason to give aid when such a relationship exists *and* when it would not be inconsistent with the provider's own conception of the good. Our challenge here, then, is somewhat more manageable than the broader discussions concerning the duty to aid: We do not need to appeal to a *substantive* moral foundation for our justification of a duty to aid within our liberal framework, but rather need only to demonstrate that a duty to aid is derived from the role one assumes as a health care professional standing in a special relationship and to do so in a manner that is not inconsistent with the negative liberty-rights of health care professionals.

Our first task is to establish what is meant by the term *beneficence*. Much common usage appeals to a substantive moral position. Beneficence, broadly speaking, concerns promotion of the patient's welfare. But because a liberal framework lacks a privileged conception of the good by which the welfare of a patient might be assessed absent the patient's own definition of this through the values *she* adopts, our understanding of beneficence centers on promotion of the patient's wishes, which define the conception of welfare to be promoted.

We have seen that once the physician-patient relationship is established, the physician takes on certain responsibilities not to "abandon" the patient. That is, she is obliged to treat for as long as the patient's condition requires it. The physician also has an obligation to recognize informed consent, stemming from a respect for patient autonomy and the patient's reserved role of assessing the benefits and burdens of treatment according to values she adopts for herself.

Both of these duties (as well as other duties toward the patient incumbent on the physician) reflect an understanding of the physician's role within a physician-patient relationship as, by nature, a role with beneficence as a core feature. This can be seen in the profession's self-understanding, as reflected in professional codes. Thus, beneficence as a core feature of the physician's role is reflected in both society's understanding of that role (as evident in the legal requirements to recognize informed consent and not to abandon the patient) and the profession's self-understanding of its role.

David is admitted to the hospital burn unit with severe burns covering most of his body. As he slowly recovers, the staff learn that these burns were sustained as a result of David's attempt to kill his wife and children by setting fire to their house while they were asleep. The repugnance of this act leads the health care staff to perceive no value in promoting this patient's health and to question their obligation to provide continued care.

The duty not to abandon can be taken as a duty of beneficence only toward a patient in need: a recognition that when a patient's condition presents a health care need, that patient's physician is expected to attend that need. Conspicuously absent in this requirement is an expectation that the physician herself will benefit. Of course, it is unlikely that a physician would be inclined to "abandon" a patient when treatment of that patient would, on balance, benefit the physician. The protection from abandonment is, in most cases, needed precisely when continued treatment would offer no benefit to the physician. The prohibition against this, then—a protection that does not require benefit but mere lack of significant "cost" to the physician — can only be taken to reflect a duty of beneficence toward the patient. It concerns a recognition that health care relationships are patient oriented and involves the promotion of welfare of those with disease or illness (at least to some degree, though I would argue that the promotion of welfare is at its core).

This broad purpose, however, and the duty of beneficence it gives rise to, is limited. It does not require the provider to promote *any* understanding of welfare. Most notably, providers are not required to promote a conception of welfare which is inconsistent with their own fundamental values and beliefs (here, a right of conscience is recognized); indeed, this limitation identifies the significance of "costs" imposed. Even where rights of conscience are exercised, it remains important that this relationship, by its very nature, involves the promotion of the patient's welfare as the patient defines it; where this involves insignificant or no cost to the provider, she may not abandon this task (the exercise of a right of conscience is *not* abandonment).

The duty to recognize informed consent reflects a concern with benefit to the patient. As we have seen, assessment of "benefit" and "burden" is in part a normative assessment. The patient reserves the role of providing the values that form the framework for making these assessments. Failure to respect this role not only might result in a failure to benefit the patient but also might harm the patient if values inconsistent with the patient's values are imposed on the patient.

Even where potential harm is not threatened, the patient is able to choose among options, all of which she might take to benefit her, by determining that one option benefits her more. The physician in this case may not override the patient's decision or impose a different treatment simply because the physician takes a different option to be preferable. (As we will see in the next chapter, this does not mean that the physician has a duty to do *anything* the patient requests; however, it does limit the types of reasons for which the physician might refuse to provide treatment.) The physician's duty to respect this choice is grounded in a duty to benefit the patient.

This social understanding of the physician's role in terms of beneficence is affirmed by the profession's self-understanding. Consider this statement from the American Medical Association's Council on Ethical and Judicial

Affairs: "The principle of patient autonomy requires that competent patients have the opportunity to choose among medically indicated treatments and to refuse any unwanted treatment. Absent countervailing obligations, physicians must respect patient's decisions" (1992, 230). The AMA also recognizes a duty of nonabandonment (1994a, xxxiv, point 5), and indeed, the preamble of the American Medical Association's "Principles of Medical Ethics" begins by stating that "the medical profession has long subscribed to a body of ethical statements developed primarily for the benefit of the patient" (1994b, xiv).

Beneficence, then, is understood as a core feature of the physician-patient relationship. This can be seen in both society's understanding of the physician-patient relationship and the profession's self-understanding. The duty of beneficence establishes a positive duty not to abandon a patient, and through this a positive duty to treat those in need. A duty to aid developed along these lines contains two features that must be present if this duty is to be consistent with a liberal framework. First, the duty cannot be applied generally but must be restricted to circumstances in which a "special relationship"—a relationship that involves the promotion of the patient's welfare (as the health care relationship does)—has been established. Second, such a duty must be restricted to conditions of insignificant or no "cost"—that is, it must preserve a provider's right of conscience to refuse to participate in the promotion of conceptions of the good inconsistent with her own fundamental values and beliefs.

Conclusion

Beneficence is important to our understanding of the professional obligations of health care providers once a relationship is established with a patient, and through this grounds a minimal duty to treat. While the duties derived from beneficence will be minimalistic (although individual physicians may conceive of themselves, on the basis of their substantive moral convictions, as having more extensive duties), beneficence does provide a justification for the positive duty to provide aid when the costs to providers are minimal.

A liberal society can establish a minimal duty to treat, even absent acceptance of Feinberg's argument that positive duties per se are no more a threat to the liberal framework than negative duties, if two important features are present. First, the duty cannot be applied generally but must be restricted to circumstances in which a "special relationship," one that involves promotion of another individual's welfare, is present. I have argued that the physician-patient relationship is such a "special relationship." Second, the duty must be restricted to circumstances where there is insignificant, or even no "cost," imposed on the person who is required to aid. This restriction requires the recognition of the health care provider's right of conscience.

6

RIGHTS OF CONSCIENCE IN THE
PHYSICIAN-PATIENT RELATIONSHIP

PROFESSIONAL LIFE IN A LIBERAL constitutional society involves a balancing of values between professional and client. This is commonly accomplished through negotiation, but in some areas of life the values in question are so fundamental and important that negotiated compromise is difficult, if not impossible. This is especially true in health care, where the values at stake involve issues of life and death and the basic capacities and abilities that give meaning to people's lives. Because health care touches on profound issues of life, death, and the quality of life, its practice can at times call for participation in activities that some health care professionals might find morally inappropriate. Requests for physician-assisted suicide, abortion, euthanasia, and the withdrawal or withholding of life support are just a few examples of controversial issues that leave little room for compromise.

As recognition of the rights of patient self-determination becomes more pervasive and patient values assume a more prominent role in formulating health care treatment plans, it is inevitable that conflicts between the values of patients and those of health care providers will increase. Much attention has been paid to patients' right to refuse treatment and to choose among various treatment options. It is also important to reflect on how to protect appropriately the health care provider's values when these conflict with the patient's. In protecting a patient's right to choose a course of treatment, we must be careful not to hold the health care professional "hostage" to the patient's values by forcing the provision of services that would not otherwise be offered, simply because the patient holds certain beliefs or values. If we do not recognize this concern, we risk forcing a health care professional—only because she has undertaken a certain profession—to engage in activities that she finds morally reprehensible.

Protection is also required for a professional's value system in our understanding of her professional role. By "professional role," I mean the conception of the activities in which the professional engages as a health care professional. Below, when I discuss allowing room for the professional to frame her role, I am concerned to let that professional's values influence the range of her work activities. We must account for how obligations attached to a professional role can be consistent with individuals *within that profession* holding different fundamental values and beliefs.

To motivate our examination of rights of conscience, let us consider the following case:

A Jehovah's Witness needs a surgical procedure or he will die. He is willing to undergo the procedure *if* he can be assured that blood products will not be used. In nine out of ten cases, the procedure does not require blood products, but the surgeon refuses to perform the procedure unless she has the option of using blood products. The surgeon acknowledges that although she *could* perform the procedure without blood products, she believes the additional risk to the patient imposed by removing the option of their use is great.

A common approach in this scenario is to allow the professional to "transfer care" of a patient when she has moral problems concerning treatment choices. I find it acceptable, in principle, to have such a policy as an ideal, to be employed *after* settling questions about *when* a right of conscience may be exercised and to be used to outline procedures for when a right of conscience *is* exercised. Before addressing these procedural questions, we must turn to questions of the nature and scope of such rights and of the types of issues over which such rights may be exercised, matters that have been largely ignored in the literature on rights of conscience in health care

It is not clear that a policy of transfer of care is always acceptable, for example, because it fails to consider adequately when a right of conscience may appropriately be exercised and the effect of the transfer of care on a patient's access to care. Allowing "unlimited" transfer of care leaves open the possibility of discriminatory practices and a transfer that may be contrary to the patient's best interests. Even though a transfer leaves the patient with access to care, it is not access to the *same care* he would have had were he to hold different values. This can be very important. Perhaps the physician who refuses to go ahead with the procedure is the most skilled at performing it, so that the patient is left with access to only inferior care. Or perhaps the patient is simply less comfortable with the "unknown" (to him) alternative physician. Transfer of care would constitute a limitation in access that is also relevant.

Even if transfer were arranged to another surgeon who was just as good, and the patient had no special attachment to the surgeon who refused to go ahead with the procedure, a sense of discrimination remains possible. The strategy of "separate but equal" to address discrimination no longer is acceptable in our society. For example, as a restaurant owner I may not deny you access to my services on certain grounds, even if I can refer you to a restaurant next door that offers the same menu. Similarly, we should be concerned about the appropriateness of denying access to health care services on certain grounds (e.g., race or religious beliefs), even if similar care remains available. At the very least, this calls for a closer examination of rights of conscience.

When disagreements over values arise between patients and health care providers, it is sometimes appropriate for the health care provider to exercise a right of conscience, and there are other times when what is called for is "tolerance." The concept of *tolerance* is crucial to a liberal constitutional society. It does not require that we advocate the aims and pursuits of others or even wish them well. It requires only that we allow others to pursue what they have chosen to pursue, consistent with the political rights of other individuals in a liberal society. We do not "tolerate" that which we advocate; we "tolerate" that with which we disagree but recognize others' rights to engage in (a child does not "tolerate" receiving Christmas presents from her parents; what the child "tolerates," rather, are things like the parents' ability to set curfews). Identifying when a right of conscience should be exercised and when tolerance is in order is of fundamental importance to the physician-patient relationship.

The nature and scope of a right of conscience is mostly avoided in discussions of rights of conscience in health care because the discussions tend to focus on the social implications of rights of conscience for issues surrounding access to care broadly conceived. For example, much has been written on the effect that rights of conscience might have on access to abortion. Articles have outlined the problems in regions of Australia and California, where rights of conscience have been so widely exercised within institutions that abortions are in effect unavailable (see Dresser 1994; Cannold 1994; Meyers and Woods 1996). While these issues are important in their own right, the social implications cannot be asserted as arguments against rights of conscience without first understanding the nature and scope of such rights. Where they apply, rights are often viewed, in the words of Ronald Dworkin, as "trumps" over considerations of social utility (see R. Dworkin 1977).

Without first establishing the nature and scope of a right of conscience, we cannot accurately identify the array of areas where such a right of might pose problems. Where a right of conscience cannot be appropriately exercised, issues of access do not arise. Only after we have established the nature and scope of a right of conscience, can we begin a discussion about how broader access issues might be addressed within our health care system.

Our challenge, then, is twofold: (1) to offer a model of the nature and scope of a right of conscience in health care which takes seriously the rights of patients to determine their lives according to values they adopt for themselves; and (2) to recognize these same rights for health care professionals, who should not lose the right of self-determination and be held to the patient's values, simply because they have entered the health care profession.

A Model for Rights of Conscience in Health Care

The model I offer as a framework for understanding rights of conscience in health care will be built on the idea that a professional's conception of her role is constrained by the broader social and political structures within which that profession is practiced. In particular, one's understanding of one's professional role must be consistent with the rights granted to individuals by a liberal constitutional society, especially the patient's right to shape decisions through evaluations that reflect her own values and beliefs. To use a somewhat extreme (but for this reason clear and noncontroversial) "twist" on the abortion example, a professional could not understand her role in such a way that she could take it on herself unilaterally to engage in activities that addressed the problem of overpopulation (which is often considered a *health* issue) by performing abortions on patients without their consent.

At the same time, it is essential to protect a professional's moral conscience within the context of her professional obligations and not to make this a function of social utility. A liberal society is concerned with protecting an individual's moral conscience. You do not lose these protections when you become a health care professional, and professionals in general should not be required to offer services that conflict with their own moral or religious beliefs.

The exercise of a right of conscience in health care should be limited to objections to the *type* of activity in question. It should not be an option when the professional disagrees with a patient about the relative (to other options) desirability of an activity to which the professional does not object in type. This is how we understand the exercise of a right of conscience in law under our liberal constitutional political system. In brief, consider one simple example: conscientious objection to fighting in a war. We live in a political system that recognizes a right of conscientious objection to fighting in a war; this can excuse one from, for instance, being drafted. But the exercise of this right is not unrestricted. Although you may exercise a right of conscience on the grounds that war is contrary to your religious beliefs, you cannot base your objections on finding this *particular* war to be a bad idea. Conscientious objection must be exercised to war in principle, not on the basis of the pros and cons of a particular instantiation of war.

To better understand this distinction in the context of health care, let us examine two scenarios in which a physician might refuse services to an individual. In the first, a physician restricts access to services *normally offered* on the basis of moral views unrelated to the treatment or procedure. For example, the physician objects to providing aggressive but exspensive treatments to a patient who is severely mentally retarded because she believes this patient's quality of life is not worth the expenditure. This raises issues concerning the role we allow for personal moral judgments in the context of social interactions and structures. The physician holds particular moral

views concerning the quality of life for a given patient. The basis of her objection is a judgment of the worth of that patient's life; were the patient not
severely retarded, she would not hesitate to provide the services.

In contrast, imagine a physician who refuses to provide abortions because
her personal moral convictions regard abortion as murder (and she does not
accept patient visits for this purpose).* Here, the physician is refusing to
offer certain services because they involve what she views as immoral acts.
In this scenario, the physician makes no judgment concerning the worth of
the (potential) patient's life or well-being but rather judges the morality of
the acts required by the procedure the patient seeks.

This distinction of type might seem clouded in some cases, as when a
Roman Catholic doctor agrees to perform abortion when the mother's life is
in danger but otherwise refuses such services. At first glance it might seem
that the doctor does not object to abortion in *type*, but this need not be the
case. The doctrine of double effect, for example, might be used to define the
act through the intention of the doctor: if the mother's life is in danger,
the procedure is to "save the mother's life"; when the mother's life is not in
danger, the procedure is defined as "killing the fetus" (which is a foreseen
but *unintended* side effect according to this doctrine). Thus, just as killing
when it is necessary to save one's own life (self-defense) is considered different in *type* from murder, the Roman Catholic doctor might reasonably
see these examples as different types of cases. (I discuss the role of circumstances in defining *type* below.)†

By focusing on the type of procedure rather than on some evaluation of
the effects or benefits for a particular patient, we exclude as a proper basis
for exercising a right of conscience an assessment that this treatment is "less
than optimal," or that in the professional's view the burdens outweigh the
benefits, or that the professional objects to the provision of services to a *particular* individual. Rather, the legitimate basis for exercising a right of conscience centers around the *type of activity*, maintaining that the type is
inconsistent with the professional's understanding of her role as a health care
professional.

---

* I use abortion throughout only as a paradigm case over which rights of conscience
are exercised. I am *not* taking a position on the abortion debate itself.

† For more on the doctrine of double effect, see Aulisio 1997.

Type versus Content

For one physician, his role as a health care professional requires that he provide the optimal medical treatment, with *optimal* defined in statistical terms. He views a patient who chooses "less effective" treatments as uncooperative and claims that he cannot in good conscience participate in that patient's poor treatment choice knowing that a better choice could have been made. He feels he must, therefore, either demand that the patient accept his recommendation or transfer the patient to the care of another physician.

Alas, many will recognize this case of the "narrow physician" as probably the most common scenario in which issues of conscience are raised—although perhaps not always exercised (they are often raised in subtle ways, as when a patient is pressured to undertake recommended treatments through the physician's threat to exercise his right of conscience). Here, the physician does not object to the type of procedure itself. Rather, *in his judgment* this procedure is less effective than an alternative. (For the purposes of discussion and illustration, I assume that the alternative treatment is an activity to which he objects not in principle but because a "more effective" alternative is possible.)

This immediately raises questions concerning patient autonomy and informed consent. Fear of abandonment, for example, can lead a patient to acquiesce to others, calling into question the legitimacy of consent. In a hospital setting this is especially important, for patients are by definition sick, vulnerable, and largely dependent on others (particularly on their health care providers).* Indeed, those who work in a clinical setting would agree that where this threat of transfer is employed, patients often—I would even go so far as to say usually[†]—acquiesce to the physician's wishes out of fear of abandonment.

---

* For a good discussion of threats and their implications for consent, see Faden and Beauchamp 1986, esp. chap. 10.

[†] Although I do not have empirical data to support this, in a real sense such data would not affect the strength of my arguments. For where we are concerned with patients' rights, the violation (or even possible violation) of such a right is wrong no matter its frequency (violating the right to refuse a ventilator is wrong whether this right is violated once or in many cases). Protection against violation of a right is provided whether or not the violation ever occurs in practice.

The "narrow physician" in my example, in defining a *type* of procedure through statistical effectiveness, raises questions about how we might define the type of procedure or treatment in the context of rights of conscience in health care. Surely *type* is in part defined by the circumstances surrounding the use of a procedure. Any given procedure may be appropriate in type for a patient in a particular medical condition, whereas it would be unsuitable for a patient who lacks this condition. For example, removal of a lung may be appropriate for a patient who has lung cancer but not for a patient who is free of that disease. It is consistent for a health care professional to view the removal of a lung in the absence of cancer as "mutilation," in a way in which the removal of the lung from a patient with cancer is not (owing to a difference in type), even though in both cases the outcome is the same—a missing lung. Note that the nature of the procedure itself is in part defined by whether it is indicated by the patient's condition.

As this approach demonstrates, to leave the criteria for type unmitigated threatens to collapse the practical and conceptual distinction between type and merit, as merit might simply be incorporated into our understanding of type. The physician's conception of his role fails to appreciate the need to incorporate the patient's values into an assessment of treatment outcomes. In the case of removing a lung, defining the procedure in type as different when cancer is present from when it is not rests on a notion of "medically indicated," which is a more basic concept than "medically optimal." This distinction is important, for "medically optimal" involves judgments about the relative desirability of treatment, whereas "medically indicated" does not. Many different treatment approaches may be "medically indicated," some of which are clearly less effective, statistically, than others.

Determining whether a procedure is indicated, unlike a judgment about relative (to other treatment options) effectiveness, may partly define the nature of the procedure without threatening a patient's ability to evaluate treatment outcomes. A judgment of "medically indicated" simply relates the treatment or procedure to the patient's condition. Even when a patient refuses the treatment, it continues to be "medically indicated" (though not "morally" or "politically" indicated given the patient's right to refuse). Judging the treatment not to be medically indicated is to define the treatment as outside the scope of medical practice, and thus outside the health care provider's "professional role."

Where a judgment that a treatment is undesirable concerns relative benefits ("it is not medically optimal"), the procedure itself may not be contrary to the professional's role. (If it is contrary to the physician's role—i.e., it is not "medically indicated"—a right of conscience could be exercised without reference to its "relative" benefits, for the alternatives are themselves of a type not consistent with the professional's role). We might ask, as a test, whether the procedure would be performed if an alternative was not available. The "narrow physician" does not object to the patient's preferred treatment per se (again, if he does, it is for reasons other than disagreement over treatment choice or the choice of a less statistically effective treatment), and he would indeed use this treatment if the more statistically effective alternative were not available. What gives rise to the physician's objection is his judgment that care is more effective through a treatment other than that chosen by the patient. This judgment of "more effective," however, not his to make; rather, in a liberal society it is reserved for the patient.

The obligations imposed by the broader liberal society, which serve as the context within which health care is practiced, constrain how the health care professional might conceive of her role and her conceptual understanding of the types of activities pursued in this role. Recognition of this broader obligation is explicit in a statement issued by the American Medical Association's Council on Ethical and Judicial Affairs: "The principle of patient autonomy requires that competent patients have the opportunity to choose among medically indicated treatments and to refuse any unwanted treatment. Absent countervailing obligations, physicians must respect patients' decisions" (1992, 2230).

It is not the mere fact that an obligation to respect patient autonomy is present in the professional codes of physicians, or even in law, which provides the great strength we attach to this obligation (though these do grant weight). Instead, there are strong moral and political reasons for this obligation, especially in a society like ours, in which no substantive moral perspective holds a "privileged" position.

As I have argued, patients retain the political right to frame the assessment of benefits and burdens of treatment according to values they adopt for themselves. Allowing *type* to be defined by "statistical effectiveness" (relative to other treatment options) ignores the possibility of other value frameworks for assessing appropriate treatment and threatens to impose this framework as the only one through which benefits and burdens might be evaluated. This runs counter to the political rights of patients. Just as you do not have the right to behave generally in a manner inconsistent with the political rights of others, you may not conceive of your professional role in a way that interferes with others' rights.

What is key is that health care practiced in a liberal society *requires* the recognition of the patient's participation in establishing the values that frame the assessment of treatment appropriateness. In this, a patient's choice or refusal of treatment (here I treat these as structurally the same)* reflects a *definition* of the effect that health care treatment will have on the patient's quality of life: the patient's decision is the framework within which any assessment of outcomes should be interpreted.

Thus, the practice of health care in a liberal society cannot allow a professional's understanding of her role to ignore patient values in assessing the effects of treatment. In this way, a liberal society places limits how a professional's values and beliefs may frame her conception of her professional role, and it restricts the considerations on which she may properly exercise a right of conscience.

The rights granted on the basis of patient autonomy are not without limits. Each individual is reserved the right to live her life according to values she adopts for herself (as long as she does not harm others in doing so). What one person believes is morally required may be seen by another as morally prohibited (e.g., the person who believes that overpopulation must be addressed through abortion will see abortion as required, while a Roman Catholic will see it as prohibited). This results in the protection of one person's "right" to do what others might see as "morally wrong" (see Waldron 1981). A person's right to live her life according to her own values, however, must be constrained by what is required of others to promote these values.

---

* A choice represents rejection of other alternatives in light of the preferred alternative. In effect, a patient's rejection of a recommended treatment recasts the range of alternatives and options available. The medically indicated options might originally consist of A, B, C, and D. Among these, the physician may recommend A. Once the patient has rejected A, it is removed *from* the *set of* available options. That set now consists of B, C, and D. The patient may subsequently reject C and D, leaving B as the only medically indicated option available. As long as B is among the set of medically indicated options, this choice by the patient should be respected.

Even though the political and social context will limit the ways in which a professional might understand her role, room must be left for exercise of the professional's own moral conscience.

A patient with end-stage cancer, who has no hope of recovery or even of leaving the hospital, is in extreme pain. He requests that the attending physician perform euthanasia, as he feels death is the only relief from pain and suffering available to him. When his request is refused, the patient asks that he at least be given the means to end his life himself, by the physician providing drugs of a type and quantity that will kill him. Again, the physician refuses, saying that he is willing to provide whatever pain relief he can, but not of a type or quantity that will cause death.

In this case, the patient claims that his quality of life is such that death would be an improvement in his condition, as it would remove him from an existence of extreme pain. Some would argue that an activity designed to bring about death in such circumstances is legitimate. Others, perhaps on the basis of particular religious or moral beliefs, do not see this as an acceptable activity. Although the health care professional has an obligation to recognize the patient's right to frame the evaluation of the effects of treatment, this does not translate to a right to frame the professional's role as requiring that she engage in a type of activity, such as bringing about death, which is inconsistent with her own moral conscience. The professional must be allowed to determine what is consistent with her conscience, even if her decision is that procedures designed to bring about death are not a type in which it is proper for her to engage.

The objection in the "euthanasia case" to a procedure or treatment on grounds of type allows the patient to retain the right to frame the evaluation of the effects of treatment. The professional might even agree that death would be preferable but still object to participating in the procedure or treatment in question because of the nature of the activity required to bring about this outcome. Recall that in the "narrow physician" case, I specified that the grounds of objection were not the nature of the treatment chosen, but that the chosen treatment was one with, in the *physician's* judgment, less desirable outcomes. Considerations of the relative (to other treatment options) benefit or burdens of treatment, as we have seen, involve the effect of treatment on the patient's quality of life and are properly framed by the patient's values. Considerations of the type of procedure in question, however, affect the professional's proper role, as they concern whether this type of activity is properly engaged in by a health care professional.

This brings me to an ambiguity within the conceptual framework I have outlined. Is it not true that recognition of a refusal of life support might be viewed as similar in type to euthanasia? That is, some might view recognizing a patient's refusal of life-sustaining treatment as an act of omission and, not morally different in type from a positive act of euthanasia (see Rachels 1975). There is in fact tremendous controversy over whether a distinction between active and passive euthanasia must collapse (see Rachels 1975; Brock 1992). I argue that a distinction must be drawn between requests and refusals in the context of rights of conscience. This distinction, however, rests not on a moral distinction between acts and omissions but rather on a political understanding of rights to adopt values for oneself and on how a distinction between requests and refusals is necessary to understand these rights while maintaining a viable conception of autonomy.

Consider again the elderly patient who prefered a shorter life in which she could continue to work in her garden to a longer life spent caring for her "brat" grandchildren (see chapter 2) and who refused surgery on this basis. Here, the patient's decision represents an evaluation that an earlier death would be preferable to life with the handicaps that would result from the surgery, and this is based on her assessment of her "quality of life" with the handicaps in question.* As we have seen, failure to recognize her right to frame the evaluation of the effects of treatment might inhibit her pursuit of *her* aims and values and actually *reduce* her quality of life.

When the evaluation that death is preferable results in a *request* for a procedure (such as euthanasia), another dimension comes into play. The patient's judgment then frames not only the evaluation of the effect of treatment on

---

* This understanding of refusals is often illegitimately conflated with requests (e.g., a request to be "left alone"), creating substantial confusion about the nature of patients' rights in certain cases. See Gert, Bernard, and Mongielnicki 1994 for a good discussion of this confusion and resulting misconceptions. An understanding of requests and refusals in terms of what judgment each frames should help to make this distinction less confusing.

her quality of life but also the professional's role, by requiring the professional to engage in a particular activity. The request would impose the patient's values on the health care professional if as a result the professional were required to engage in the activities requested. Clearly, requiring that one person's *requests* always be recognized can pose a direct threat to another person's values. The rights granted to individuals in a liberal society do not allow one person to require others to assume a positive role in promoting his or her own values or goals.*

The balance of rights in a society that seeks to protect each individual's conscience must recognize a distinction between a requirement to assume a positive role in achieving the aims of others and the toleration of alternative values and aims. Without this distinction, autonomy of conscience is not possible (see Hart 1962). As we have seen, we do not tolerate that which we advocate; we tolerate that with which we disagree. If we do not recognize refraining from a forced inhibition of another's pursuit of aims with which we disagree (a minimal conception of toleration) as being distinct from actively promoting those aims, we are forced to allow, in a society that seeks to protect each individual's conscience, pursuit of *only* those aims to which *nobody* objects (and tolerance of those aims would be tantamount to forced pursuit of them). The concept of autonomy in such a society would be hollow at best.

Requests and refusals (or choice from among alternatives, which I take here as similar in structure to refusals, as both represent an assessment of burdens and benefits) pose structural differences in terms of the imposition of values. A patient's refusal is an evaluation that treatment does not offer effects that are a net benefit. Likewise, a choice from among alternative treatments is an evaluation that the alternative selected offers the most beneficial effects. Importantly, the professional is not asked in these instances to engage in an activity that might be seen as inconsistent with her understanding of her role. Rather, she is asked to refrain from a procedure or to pursue an alternative procedure; she is not to impose on the patient her own values and beliefs about how to evaluate the relative effects of treatment. (Remem-

---

* I leave open here whether a request for assistance with dying is appropriate. Instead, my focus is on why it *might* be appropriate to exercise a right of conscience over such a request (and how this differs from refusals).

ber that I assume the alternative treatment is not itself of a type inconsistent with the professional's values, but rather is seen by the professional as "less effective" than other alternatives.) The patient does not frame the professional's role, only the evaluation of the effects of treatment on her own conception of her quality of life. Thus, not to allow a refusal (or choice) threatens to impose the professional's conception of the purpose of health care on the patient.*

To require a health care professional to recognize the patient's right to frame the evaluation of outcomes is not to impose the patient's values on the health care professional. It is simply to acknowledge that in our society a profession is practiced in the context of standards that evaluate outcomes differently for different individuals; that is, a society like ours (which protects an individual's right to define her own quality of life) demands that the specific standards that evaluate the effects of treatment on a particular individual's quality of life be provided by that individual. To require the health care professional's recognition of patient autonomy does not impose a conception of a professional role on the professional; it acknowledges a context within which the pursuit of a given professional purpose (for example, improving or restoring the patient's quality of life) must be understood.

Requests, in contrast, frame not only the evaluation of the effects of treatment but also the professional's role. The particular activity required by the requested procedure may or may not be consistent with the professional's conception of her role. Although the professional has an obligation to recognize patient autonomy in evaluating the effects of treatment, this obligation does not extend to recognizing the patient's conception of the professional's role by requiring the professional to engage in *any* type of activity requested by the patient. It is appropriate, then, to ask whether the role indicated by the requested procedure is consistent with the professional's understanding of her role. The professional's own fundamental values and beliefs may place constraints on the types of activities in which she may engage, and thus frame her conception of her role as a health care professional. Not to allow this is to threaten to impose the patient's values on the health care professional.

---

* For a good discussion of the different requirements that arise from requests and refusals, especially in the context of the strict requirement to respect refusals and less strict requirement to carry out requests, see Gert, Bernard, and Mongielnicki 1994.

In short, on the one hand, a request that is inconsistent with a professional's conception of her role might impose the patient's values and beliefs on the professional (in the absence of a right of conscience); on the other hand, objection to a patient's refusal or choice among alternatives (consistent in type with the professional's understanding of her role) threatens to impose a professional's values on the patient. For this reason, we need to recognize both the obligation of health care professionals to frame evaluation of the effects of treatment on a patient's quality of life in terms of the patient's values and the right of the professional to frame her role as a health care professional in the context of her own values.

Rights of conscience are designed to protect exactly this balance. Indeed, this model is consistent with our understanding of rights of conscience more generally, as well as rights protecting freedom in society in general. Such rights protect an individual from the imposition of others' values in determining the desirability of an action in terms of the action's effect on the individual's quality of life, but they do not allow an individual to force others to engage in activities that are inconsistent with *their* fundamental values and beliefs.

Conclusion

Recall that in the example that motivated the examination of rights of conscience at the beginning of this chapter, the surgeon acknowledged that the procedure *could* be done without the use of blood products, but she viewed as a poor decision the additional risk that prohibiting this option posed. We saw that it was not the *type* of procedure to which the surgeon objected. It is even likely that were the use of blood products not a technological possibility, the surgeon would go ahead with the procedure, given the certainty of death if the procedure were not performed. The patient's refusal of blood products is a judgment concerning the benefits of this therapy. The patient balanced the potential benefit from receiving this therapy for his continued life in this world against the belief that receiving blood products would result in eternal damnation; the balance was clearly in favor of refusal. Although the surgeon disagrees with the patient about his beliefs, the patient retains the right to structure his life according to her own values and beliefs. In this, the surgeon's objection looks similar to that of our "narrow physician."

Rights of conscience in health care must be exercised in the context of patients' rights to informed consent. This requires that we acknowledge limits on the exercise of rights of conscience. We must respect the patient's right ultimately to judge whether a potential therapy, treatment, or procedure offers appropriate benefits, while simultaneously recognizing that this does not translate to a right to demand anything that the patient might view as beneficial.

What if the balance of benefits and burdens of our case were not so clearly defined? For example, what if the patient had a reasonable chance of recovery without surgery (though not great—for the sake of argument, we will say approximately a 20 percent chance of recovery)? Suppose also that surgery *with* blood products would increase the patient's chances for recovery such that he would have a 50 percent chance of recovery rather than 20 percent. Surgery *without* the use of blood products, however, would reduce the benefits of surgery, say, to 35 percent. Our model tells us that judging the value of this increased chance of recovery in the context of one's life overall is reserved for the patient.

For a right of conscience to be justified, the risks associated with surgery performed without the option to use blood products would have to become great enough that surgery was not "medically indicated." If performing surgery without blood products were of greater risk to the patient than not performing surgery at all, the physician might justifiably exercise a right of conscience on the grounds that surgery in these circumstances is not medically indicated. Here, the physician's objection is based not on a disagreement with the patient over the value of using blood products but on the appropriate use of medical technique—that is, that the procedure is not indicated in circumstances in which the risks of surgery are greater than the risks of no surgery. The physician's conscience in defining her role is protected, but not at the expense of the patient's right to define the values that frame his life.

In my model, I have attempted to balance these concerns through two fundamental distinctions: (1) objection to the type of treatment or procedure in question is separate from objection to the patient's evaluation of benefits and risks/burdens of treatment; and (2) refusal of treatment is not the same as request for treatment. This leaves a wide range of latitude for a health care professional to exercise a right of conscience based on her values, in that those values retain a significant influence, but within the limits imposed on defining her role by the obligation to recognize the patient's right to frame the evaluation of benefits and burdens. It also captures the importance of protecting the patient's autonomy-based rights in providing the framework for assessing the effects of treatment on her quality of life.

7

CONCLUSION
Health Care Ethics Committees and Consultants in a Liberal Framework

THROUGHOUT, I HAVE FOCUSED on the implications of a liberal political and social context for bioethics decision making. Protecting an individual's right to frame the values that guide her life is, as we have seen, a fundamental concern of our liberal society. Now I will examine how the concern to respect patient autonomy has given rise to the development of health care ethics committees and consultants, and how these developments can be understood in a liberal context.

In most areas of social life, protection of individual autonomy is accomplished through a "hands-off" approach coupled with the principle of tolerance. Remember that we cannot be said to tolerate values with which we agree; rather, tolerance is necessary only for values we do not ourselves share. To tolerate these values, we need not *accept* them, but we must recognize the right of others to adopt them. This protects our right to adopt certain values with which others may disagree. In health care practice, it protects a patient's right to adopt values with which a health care provider or others may not agree.

A hands-off approach does not always suffice to protect individual autonomy. Alan Montefiore (1975, 7) offers an example of two children involved in a dispute: one is older, stronger, and more resourceful. If the children are left to their own devices, the interests of the younger, weaker child are likely to be subverted. That is, without intervention to "level the playing field," the older child's wishes will prevail. In a clinical setting, patients are vulnerable. They are by definition sick, often weak, and largely dependent on others, particularly those who provide care. Because patients are vulnerable and because remaining neutral would likely result (in cases where value differences exist between patient and health care provider) in the provider's values prevailing, it is important to provide mechanisms to protect the standing of the patient's values and to ensure that these are recognized in those areas where they should be protected. To fill this role, health care ethics committees and consultants were developed.

The Role of Health Care Ethics Committees

Health care ethics committees have developed along with our society's increased awareness of individual rights in a variety of arenas. The growth of bioethics in general began as our society reflected on a wide array of civil rights reforms needed to bring our political systems in line with our liberal ideology (and, in health care, with an increased emphasis on patient autonomy). Over the past twenty-five years, ethics committees have been advocated by the courts (*In re* Quinlan, 70 NJ 10,355 A2d 647, cert. denied, 429 US 922 [1976]), supported by a report of the President's Commission for the Study of Ethical Problems in Medicine and Biomedical and Behavioral Research (1983, 5), and even required by laws and regulations in several states (Leeman et al. 1997). The Joint Commission on Accreditation of Healthcare Organizations (JCAHO) now requires that hospitals provide some mechanism for addressing ethical conflict. As recently as the early 1980s fewer than 1 percent of hospitals had formal ethics committees, whereas surveys conducted in the early 1990s suggested that as many as 85 percent of hospitals have one (Ross et al. 1993, ix).

The functions of health care ethics committees are generally threefold: education, policy development, and case consultation (ibid., 5–6). The education function normally consists in the provision of in-service or continuing education sessions, grand rounds, or monthly forums in which hospital staff members learn about ethical issues that arise in clinical care. Topics include advance directives, surrogate decision making, and the withdrawal of life support. Education is an important first step in protecting patients' rights. Awareness of how a patient's values might influence care is often difficult, and education designed to make health care providers sensitive to this is essential.

Ethics committees are also commonly charged with developing and re-viewing institutional policy. Typically, the committee will review policies for consistency with respect to patients' rights and will recommend changes to better reflect this concern. Areas in which health care ethics committees might review institutional policies include do-not-resuscitate (DNR) orders, informed consent, advance directives, brain death and organ donation, and a myriad of other areas. As the practice of health care is reformed to better re-spect patients' rights, institutional policies, with their long history of pater-nalism, must undergo similar reform.

The most vague and controversial function of health care ethics commit-tees is ethics case consultation. At different institutions, the committees adopt different methods for providing ethics case consultation services. The three most common methods are individual consultants, consultation teams drawn from the larger health care ethics committee, and review by the entire ethics committee (SHHV-SBC 1998, 11). Regardless of the method used, the basic purpose of ethics consultation remains the same. A task force created by the Society for Health and Human Values (SHHV) and the Society for Bio-ethics Consultation (SBC)* to study standards for the practice of bioethics consultation characterized ethics consultation as follows:

> The general goal of health care ethics consultation is to: improve the pro-vision of health care and its outcome through the identification, analysis, and resolution of ethical issues as they emerge in consultation regarding particular clinical cases in health care institutions.
> This general goal is more likely to be achieved if consultation accom-plishes the intermediary goals of helping to: identify and analyze the na-ture of the value uncertainty or conflict that underlies the consultation; facilitate resolution of conflicts in a respectful atmosphere with attention to the interests, rights, and responsibilities of those involved; inform insti-tutional efforts at policy development, quality improvement, and appro-priate utilization of resources by identifying the causes of ethical problems and promoting practices consistent with ethical norms and standards; as-sist individuals in handling current and future ethical problems by pro-viding education in health care ethics. (1998, 8)

The primary goal of ethics consultation is to identify and analyze value uncertainty or conflict arising in specific clinical cases. To help understand

---

* These organizations have now merged, along with the American Association of Bioethics, to form the American Society for Bioethics and Humanities.

this role, let us consider an analogy to other forms of consultation in health care. An attending physician may be concerned with identifying and analyzing a wide range of physical, emotional, and value issues for any given patient. When one area becomes particularly complicated, she may seek help in the form of a specialist. Thus, a cardiologist may be sought for complicated cases involving the heart. Because the cardiologist works primarily in this area, she may more readily recognize features of a case that suggest a particular problem. Likewise, an ethicist may be sought when cases involve complicated values whose relevance and relationships are unclear. By helping to identify, articulate, and analyze values in the context of the issue at hand, the ethics consultant can help to address uncertainty and conflict and to protect the rights of patients in the clinical setting.

Is Ethics Consultation Consistent with a Liberal Political Framework?

The popular media have suggested that ethics case consultation may be inappropriate. Ruth Shalit, for example, criticizes ethicists for perceiving themselves as keepers of the moral truth: "More than mere advisors, these fee-for-service philosophers see themselves as experts, capable of passing judgment on what should and should not be done in matters of life and death" (1997, 24).* Shalit goes on to criticize ethicists because, she claims, they "wield 'ethics case analysis grids' with algorithmic certainty," and she says that "ethicists frequently are called on to advise on contested questions about when life should end, a type of decision they claim to be entitled to make by dint of their superior knowledge and skills. When the views of ethicists conflict with the wishes of patients and families, the ethicists may naturally be inclined to favor their own judgments: After all, who is the expert here?" (ibid.).

These concerns are present in the bioethics literature as well, in almost identical form (and terms). Giles Scofield has published several articles criticizing ethicists for their belief in the "algorithmic certainty" of moral answers, claiming that the practice of the ethicist is by nature "antidemocratic,"

---

* I would contest Shalit's characterization of ethicists as fee-for-service. At least at the medical center I am familiar with, the ethics consultation service is provided at no charge. While it may be argued that the costs are ultimately passed on to patients, the ethics staff are compensated at a fixed salary, not reimbursed on a fee-for-service basis.

and accusing ethicists of seeking inappropriate power. To be certain, the concerns expressed by Scofield and the popular media are important in that a liberal society does not recognize "expertise" over the answers to substantive moral questions, reserving this judgment to each individual in matters affecting their own life and welfare.

Ethics case consultation, however, need not take a form in which a substantive moral position is advanced and advocated. Concerns like those expressed above seem linked to a misunderstanding of the ethicist's role in the clinical setting. Specifically, the concerns seem linked to a belief that in identifying values and helping to articulate and analyze their relevance in decision making, the ethicist makes pronouncements concerning the "correctness" of the values in question. Let us consider why this is thought to be the case.

As ethics consultants proceed with identifying, articulating, and analyzing the implications of values for health care treatment decisions, it is hoped that conflicts or difficulties in determining appropriate action will be resolved. This is accomplished primarily by identifying how the values of the person who is reserved the role of providing the values that will frame this decision might influence the decision. For example, if the patient has that role, the ethics consultant will focus on the patient's values, and try to assess the implications for the determination of treatment. Thus, a recommendation is often made about appropriate treatment based upon the patient's articulated values. The problem, Shalit tells us, relates to the ethicists' failure to recognize the difference between values and science.

> The problem with all this is basic. "Clinical ethics" is not medicine, which is to say it is not science, which is to say it is to a very large degree whatever anyone wants it to be. In attempting to make a medical profession out of the study of what is morally right and wrong, ethicists confuse the empirical and theoretical. A surgeon who recommends amputation of a gangrenous limb as the right procedure means by "right" an action that will save the patient's life. What a philosopher means by "right" is the action that is most moral. But these two "rights" are not equally absolute. The surgeon's recommendation rests on an agreed-upon set of facts and criteria: there is no question that amputation is the appropriate action in extreme cases of gangrene. (1997, 24)

Shalit's claim that there is no question that amputation is the appropriate action is a strong position and might itself be a significant threat to a patient's right to refuse treatment because the physician is said to know the "right" thing to do, "medically" speaking. Remember the case of Lydia (chapter 2), who was faced with the need for surgery that could significantly extend her life but would result in (what the health care team considered) "minor" handicaps, which would inhibit her ability to work in her garden. From a medical perspective, the health care team was very confident that there was a right course of action, and this was to go ahead with surgery. To Lydia, the surgery represented a threat to the most meaningful activity in her life; a shorter life that included this activity was considered by *Lydia* to be of greater value than a longer life without this activity. The role of bioethics is precisely that of calling into question whether *any* treatment is appropriate "without question." This role involves no claim concerning the correctness of values nor prescription for what action ought to be taken. We can learn from the identification and analysis of a patient's values, without judgments concerning the truth or falsity of those values. There is no need for pronouncement concerning the "right" moral answer nor any claim to serve as "keeper of the moral truth."

Ultimately, the most serious mistake is to think that either judgment, moral or medical, concerning what treatment should be done is absolute. A view like that expressed by Shalit seems to imply a belief that there is an absolute right action from a medical perspective. Recognition that this is not so—and recognition of why it is not through an appreciation of how any judgment of "right" treatment presupposes values—is one of the primary goals of ethics consultation and an important theme of this book.

The presupposition of value is involved in subtle ways in nearly every decision made concerning appropriate treatment (especially where a variety of treatment options are available with different potential benefits and side effects; see chapter 2). This is because a judgment of "appropriate" is by nature a normative judgment. Shalit is correct in acknowledging the different uses of the term *right* in, for example, mathematics and ethics. What is in question, however, is whether "right treatment" is more like the use of "right" in mathematics than in ethics. The ethicist claims not that determinations of right treatment from a moral perspective has the algorithmic certainty of mathematics, but that determination of "right" or "appropriate" treatment is at least partly normative and thus not wholly factual. Shalit's statement that "there is no question that amputation is the appropriate action in extreme cases of gangrene" does not account for the possibility that for some patients, this may not be so. (I discussed these types of cases in detail in chapter 2.)

Deciding appropriate treatment certainly involves what resembles "factual" elements,* and these "facts" provide the primary data on which treatment decisions are made. For example, if there are simply no treatments available for a given condition, the question of whether a treatment is appropriate will not arise because of the "factual" circumstances. As well, when there are limited treatment options with stark contrast (accept surgery and probably live; do not accept surgery and surely die), identifying values and their impact may be relatively straightforward. This is not because values are not presupposed, but because the factual circumstances are such that given the limited array of options, the values of particular individuals may to a large extent converge (most people prefer to live than to die). However, even where there is but one viable treatment option from a "factual" perspective, the patient retains the right to refuse that treatment, and a judgment of "appropriate" remains partly normative, even here.

Determining "appropriate" treatment, then, is itself a determination that includes, among other things, a value judgment. As we have seen, what is right for one patient may not be right for another. Whether a given treatment is appropriate depends on whether the potential benefits of that treatment outweigh the burdens it imposes on the patient. This judgment requires that we consider the patient's perspective in assessing the benefits and burdens of treatment. To fail to do so is inconsistent with a liberal constitutional society and with the rights of patients in such a society.

Ethics case consultation can be useful, not only in protecting the rights of a patient but also in protecting a health care professional's rights of conscience. New procedures and technologies are rapidly expanding the range of conditions health care professionals are asked to address and the nature of health care intervention. Abortion, physician-assisted suicide, artificial insemination, and many emerging genetic treatments go beyond the act of simply providing care, intervening on natural processes in profound ways. As we have seen, while a patient's right to be involved in the decision-making process is essential, it should not be confused with an ability of the patient to demand any treatment or procedure.

* "Factual" is in quotes in recognition of the tremendous controversy over the nature of medical "knowledge."

Conclusion

The role of the ethics consultant is not one of advocacy per se, but of ensuring, to the extent possible, that the values and rights of all parties are recognized and respected. It is not an outcome (such as having the values of one party prevail) that is the focus of the consultant. Rather, it is the legitimacy and fairness of the process. Just as a philosopher evaluates an argument on the basis of the validity of its structure rather than on the argument's conclusion, the ethics consultant will focus on the legitimacy and fairness of the decision-making process rather than on the content of the decision per se.

There is no "absolute moral right" presupposed by ethics consultation. To the contrary, what is presupposed is that there is no privileged position by which one person's conception of "right" may be imposed on another. This is true not only in protecting the patient through informed consent but also in protecting the provider's rights of conscience in refusing to participate in procedures she finds objectionable. The ethics consultant is concerned that the values and rights of each party involved be recognized and respected. Whose values will prevail on a given issue is a function of the social and political system, not of the ethicist. A competent patient's legal right to refuse treatment, for example, is not a right that the ethicist decides the patient does or does not have. Both the right in question and the potential exceptions to the patient's ability to exercise this right are defined by the political society, not by the ethicist. This is how a liberal political framework places boundaries on bioethics decision making.

The SHHV-SBC task force recognizes these political dimensions of health care decision making: "In our society . . . ethical issues emerge against a complex background of developing health care technologies, and political, social, communal, institutional, professional and individual values. . . . These decisions must be made in a pluralistic context in which individuals have the political right, arising from the basic societal value of autonomy, to pursue their own conception of the good" (1998, 8). As well, the task force maintains that ethics consultants should not attempt to impose moral views, stating: "Ethics consultants . . . should not usurp moral decision-making authority or impose their values on other involved parties" (7).

This understanding of the ethicist's role has important implications for Scofield's claims that ethicists are by nature "antidemocratic." Scofield has argued extensively against the role of clinical ethics in health care decision making. While he recognizes some potential benefits in the clinical setting, he maintains that these benefits should be realized through education and retrospective case review rather than through participation in the decision-making process itself. His reasons for this are varied, but the core of his concerns seem to be the nature of moral expertise and the fact that such expertise is "antidemocratic." States Scofield: "Ethics is not like mathematics or the physical sciences. Value systems cannot be reduced to taxonomies, nor moral reasoning to algorithmic certainty" (1993, 420). Scofield's criticism takes up from this: "Even if we could agree about the values that should form the basis of ethical decision-making, there are no objective truths about how these values will or should be weighed by different persons in the same or different situations" (ibid.).

On this basis, Scofield further argues that: "in a democratic society, ethics is everybody's business, not the exclusive domain of a particular group. Thus, the power and authority ethics consultants seek are essentially antidemocratic" (1993, 421). This is not quite true, for several reasons. Nothing about democracy prohibits the imposition of a privileged point of view. As long as the majority agree that, for example, Christian ethics should be privileged, that ethical perspective could be imposed on the society at large, including those who are not Christian. Although it is true that in a democracy individuals are given a voice in what values are imposed in such a way, that input would be small consolation to, for instance, a Muslim living in a predominant Christian society. As one prominent political theorist, John Gray, said: "Where it is unlimited, democratic government cannot be a liberal government since it respects no domain of independence or liberty as being immune to invasion by governmental authority. Unlimited democratic government, from a liberal point of view, is rather a form of totalitarianism—the form predicted and criticized by J. S. Mill in *On Liberty*" (1986, 74).

This, however, is trifling. For I believe that what Scofield has in mind is liberal constitutionalism rather than democracy. Liberal constitutionalism protects individuals from the imposition of another individual's or group's perspective on ethics and makes ethics "everybody's business." Indeed, liberal constitutionalism is motivated in large part by concerns that democracy absent this constraint could lead to a "tyranny of the majority." Therefore, I assume that what Scofield means by "democracy" is the protections afforded by liberal constitutionalism. Although Scofield may intend to critique ethics consultation from the perspective of democracy rather than liberal constitutionalism, it is the latter that is the distinctive feature of American political society. It is from this perspective that I will devote my efforts to defend ethics consultation.

To Scofield, the nature of claims of expertise seem to pose ipso facto a threat to the "democratic"* ideal that all persons are equal: "Professional experts invariably create a tension within a democratic society, between the belief that all persons are equal and the claim that some, by virtue of special knowledge or skill, are superior to others" (1993, 421). Although it is true that liberal societies regard individuals as "equals," this is not to say that these societies believe that all persons are equally skilled, intelligent, or able in any given area. The sense of equality asserted by liberal societies is a sense of *equal standing*; that is, a political notion of equality (not a metaphysical notion about human nature) which disregards even recognized inequalities in aptitude, skill, intelligence, and other traits for political purposes. This political notion of equality is perfectly consistent with "expertise"—both professional and nonprofessional.†

As a political notion, the equality espoused by liberal societies protects a person's standing under that political system by protecting his personal authority over his own life (autonomy), regardless of his expertise or lack thereof. I may choose to consult an auto mechanic, but I am not required, politically, to follow her recommendations. Likewise, I may consult a physician because I recognize her "expertise," but then I may refuse her recommendations. One may argue about the moral, prudential, or other obligations imposed by expertise, but in a liberal constitutional society, the individual retains the right to reject expertise, and this protects individual conscience.

The political notion of equal standing is a far more important and valuable notion of equality than one that relies on a view of equal aptitudes, skills, and ability. It is a fact that individuals differ in their areas of expertise, skill, and

* I will continue to use this terminology in describing Scofield's position, even though I take Scofield's ultimate concern to be with liberal constitutionalism.

† The real problem of the "professional" lies not with "expertise," but with the act of licensing, which seems to impose a particular conception of value and allows a profession to enforce *its* ideals, and even to restrict the ability to practice (and restrict who may practice). There is, however, no such licensing for ethicists. Indeed, SHHV-SBC (1998, 31–32) recommended against licensing or certification.

aptitudes. This does not necessarily mean that I am unable to gain expertise in other areas should I choose to devote my energies toward that end, though there may well be areas in which I simply lack the abilities to excel (I strongly suspect that no amount of practice or effort would allow me to beat Michael Jordan one-on-one!). Any one individual is limited in the range of expertise that can be achieved. I may choose to spend my time learning philosophy at the cost of learning to repair my car. Because I have limited time, resources, and interests, I will gain expertise in some areas and need to rely on others who have different areas of expertise.*

The expertise of the ethics consultant lies in the identification of values that underlie specific positions, analysis of the implications of those values, and the ability to shift, at least to some degree, from one's own perspective on a particular question to the perspective that embodies another's values, and then help to articulate that perspective. These are skills that the study of normative ethics develops and that might be of use to some individuals in reaching a decision. That is, reflection on a patient's values and their relationship to the decision in question might help the patient make a decision on the basis of her own values, and it may help health care providers better understand the perspective from which "appropriate" treatment might be judged. Most significant then is that the role of the ethicist does not usurp the patient's judgment; indeed, it strengthens it.

In this way, the presence of ethics in the clinical setting—indeed, in the decision-making process itself—can help to protect patient autonomy. There is no "power" claimed, no special knowledge about the "morally right" answer. The ethicist merely offers assistance in recognizing how judgments of appropriate treatment are affected by presuppositions of value, and helps to identify and analyze values relevant to a particular decision. The ethicist does not impose a decision.

The clinical setting calls for a mechanism to protect patient autonomy in framing the evaluation of treatment according to the patient's own judgment. Health care ethics committees and consultants serve the role of providing this mechanism. Through a threefold function of education, policy

---

* This is how we live our lives, and our autonomy is largely reflected in our choices of what areas we devote our energies to and in what areas we appeal to others for help. See May 1994.

Conclusion

development, and case consultation, health care ethics committees strive to make the health care community more sensitive to the ways in which values are presupposed in the delivery of health care and to help reform the practice of health care so that the patient's values can frame treatment decisions. To accomplish this, however, it is important that health care ethics committees and consultants refrain from imposing their own values by making "pronouncements" about *the* morally right course of action or treatment. The role of health care ethics committees and consultants should be to identify, articulate, and analyze the implications of value judgments for health care treatment.

REFERENCES

Agich, George J., and Thomas May. 1997. "Paternalism, Moral Agency and Alcoholism." In Rem Edwards and Wayne Shelton (eds.), *Advances in Bioethics: Values, Ethics, and Alcoholism*. Greenwich, Conn.: JAI Press.

American Medical Association, Council on Ethical and Judicial Affairs. 1992. "Decisions Near the End of Life," *JAMA* 267:2229–33.

———. 1994a. "Fundamental Elements of the Patient-Physician Relationship." In *Code of Medical Ethics: Current Opinions and Annotations*. Chicago: American Medical Association.

———. 1994b. "Principles of Medical Ethics." In *Code of Medical Ethics: Current Opinions and Annotations*. Chicago: American Medical Association.

Annas, George. 1975. *The Rights of Hospital Patients*. New York: Avon Books.

———. 1993. *Standard of Care: The Law of American Bioethics*. New York: Oxford University Press.

Appelbaum, Paul, and Loren Roth. 1981. "Clinical Issues in the Assessment of Competency," *American Journal of Psychiatry* 138:1462–67.

Arneson, Richard J. 1990. "Neutrality and Utility," *Canadian Journal of Philosophy* 20, no. 2 (June): 215–40.

Aulisio, Mark. 1997. "One Person's *Modus Ponens*: Boyle, Absolutist Catholicism, and the Doctrine of Double Effect," *Christian Bioethics* 3:142–57.

Berlin, Isaiah. 1969. *Four Essays on Liberty*. London: Oxford University Press.

Brock, Dan. 1992. "Voluntary and Active Euthanasia," *Hastings Center Report* 22, no. 2 (March–April): 10–22.

Buchanan, Allen. 1988. "Advance Directives and the Personal Identity Problem," *Philosophy and Public Affairs* 17:277–302.

Buchanan, Allen E., and Dan W. Brock. 1989. *Deciding for Others: The Ethics of Surrogate Decision Making*. New York: Cambridge University Press.

Cannold, Leslie. 1994. "Consequences for Patients of Health Care Professionals' Conscientious Actions," *Journal of Medical Ethics* 20:80–86.

Coker, Richard J. 2000. *From Chaos to Coercion*. New York: St. Martin's Press.

Conot, Robert E. 1983. *Justice at Nuremberg*. New York: Harper & Row Publishers.

Drane, James. 1985. "The Many Faces of Competency," *Hastings Center Report* 15, no. 2 (April): 17–21.

References

———. 1994. *Clinical Bioethics*. Kansas City: Sheed and Ward.

Dresser, Rebecca. 1984. "Bound to Treatment: The Ulysses Contract," *Hastings Center Report* 14, no. 3 (June): 13–16.

———. 1994. "Freedom of Conscience, Professional Responsibility, and Access to Abortion," *Journal of Law, Medicine and Ethics* 22, no. 3: 280–85.

Dworkin, Gerald. 1974. "Non-Neutral Principles." In Norman Daniels (ed.), *Reading Rawls*. New York: Basic Books.

Dworkin, Ronald. 1977. *Taking Rights Seriously*. Cambridge, Mass.: Harvard University Press.

Elster, Jon. 1979. *Ulysses and the Sirens*. New York: Cambridge University Press.

Emanuel, Linda, Michael Barry, John Stoeckle, Lucy Ettelson, and Ezekiel Emanuel. 1991. "Advance Directives for Medical Care: A Case for Greater Use," *New England Journal of Medicine* 324:889–95.

Faden, Ruth, and Tom Beauchamp. 1986. *A History and Theory of Informed Consent*. New York: Oxford University Press.

Feinberg, Joel. 1980. *Rights, Justice, and the Bounds of Liberty*. Princeton, N.J.: Princeton University Press.

———. 1984. *Harm to Others*. New York: Oxford University Press.

———. 1985. *Offense to Others*. New York: Oxford University Press.

———. 1986. *Harm to Self*. New York: Oxford University Press.

———. 1988. *Harmless Wrongdoing*. New York: Oxford University Press.

Fetters, Michael. 1998. "The Family in Medical Decision Making: Japanese Perspectives," *Journal of Clinical Ethics* 9:132–46.

Fischer, John Martin (ed.). 1986. *Moral Responsibility*. Ithaca: Cornell University Press.

Gert, Bernard, James Bernat, and R. Peter Mongielnicki. 1994. "Distinguishing between Patients' Refusals and Requests," *Hastings Center Report* 24, no. 6 (Nov.–Dec.): 13–15.

Gray, John. 1986. *Liberalism*. Minneapolis: University of Minnesota Press.

Hall, John A., and G. John Ikenberry. 1989. *The State*. Minneapolis: University of Minnesota Press.

Hart, H. L. A. 1962. *Law, Liberty and Morality*. Stanford: Stanford University Press.

Hohfeld, W. 1964. *Fundamental Legal Conceptions*. New Haven: Yale University Press.

Hoshino, Kazumasa. 1995. "Autonomous Decision Making and Japanese Tradition," *Cambridge Quarterly of Healthcare Ethics* 4, no. 1: 71–74.

Howell, Timothy, Ronald Diamond, and Daniel Wikler. 1982. "Is There a Case for Voluntary Commitment?" In Tom Beauchamp and LeRoy Walter (eds.), *Contemporary Issues in Bioethics*. Belmont, Calif.: Wadsworth.

Kaplan, Kenneth. 1988. "Assessing Judgment," *General Hospital Psychiatry* 10, no. 3: 202–8.

LeBlang, Theodore, W. Eugene Basanta, and Robert Kane. 1996. *The Law of Medical Practice in Illinois*, 2nd ed. Rochester, N.Y.: Lawyers Cooperative Publishing.

References

Leeman, Calvin, John Fletcher, Edward Spencer, and Sigrid Fry-Revere. 1997. "Quality Control for Hospitals' Clinical Ethics Services: Proposed Standards," *Cambridge Quarterly of Healthcare Ethics* 6, no. 3: 257–68.

Lomasky, Loren. 1990. "But Is It Liberalism? A Review of Raz's *The Morality of Freedom*," *Critical Review* 4:86–105.

Lynn, Joanne, and Joan M. Teno. 1993. "After the Patient Self-Determination Act: The Need for Empirical Research on Formal Advance Directives," *Hastings Center Report* 23, no. 1 (Jan.–Feb.): 20–24.

May, Thomas. 1993. "The Nurse under Physician Authority," *Journal of Medical Ethics* 19:223–27.

———. 1994. "The Concept of Autonomy," *American Philosophical Quarterly* 31: 133–44.

———. 1997a. "On Raz and the Obligation to Obey the Law," *Law and Philosophy* 16:19–36.

———. 1997b. "Reassessing the Reliability of Advance Directives," *Cambridge Quarterly of Healthcare Ethics* 6, no. 3: 325–38.

———. 1998. *Autonomy, Authority, and Moral Responsibility*. Dordrecht, The Netherlands: Kluwer Academic Publishers.

McClennen, Edward F. 1990. *Rationality and Dynamic Choice*. New York: Cambridge University Press.

McIntyre, Alison. 1994. "Guilty Bystanders? On the Legitimacy of Duty to Rescue Statutes," *Philosophy and Public Affairs* 23:157–91.

Meyers, Christopher, and Robert Woods. 1996. "An Obligation to Provide Abortion Services: What Happens When Physicians Refuse?" *Journal of Medical Ethics* 22:115–20.

Mill, John Stuart. 1956. *On Liberty*. Indianapolis: Bobbs-Merrill.

Montefiore, Alan. 1975. *Neutrality and Impartiality*. New York: Cambridge University Press.

Nagel, Thomas. 1979. "Moral Luck." In Thomas Nagel (ed.), *Mortal Questions*. New York: Cambridge University Press.

Ohio State Bar Association and Ohio State Medical Association. 1991. "Advanced Directives for Health Care: Standard Forms." Special Insert to *Ohio Lawyer* (Sept./Oct.).

President's Commission for the Study of Ethical Problems in Medicine and Biomedical and Behavioral Research. 1983. *Deciding to Forgo Life-Sustaining Treatment*. Washington, D.C.: U.S. Government Printing Office.

Rachels, James. 1975. "Active and Passive Euthanasia," *New England Journal of Medicine* 292:78–80.

Radden, Jennifer. 1992. "Planning for Mental Disorder: Buchanan and Brock on Advance Directives," *Social Theory and Practice* 18, no. 2: 165–86.

Rawls, John. 1971. *A Theory of Justice*. Cambridge, Mass.: Harvard University Press.

———. 1985. "Justice as Fairness: Political, not Metaphysical," *Philosophy and Public Affairs* 14, no. 2: 223–51.

References

Raz, Joseph. 1978. "Reasons for Action, Decisions, and Norms." In Joseph Raz (ed.), *Practical Reasoning*. New York: Oxford University Press.

———. 1986. *The Morality of Freedom*. New York: Oxford University Press.

———. 1990. *Practical Reason and Norms*. Princeton, N.J.: Princeton University Press.

Richards, David A. J. 1982. *Sex, Drugs, Death, and the Law*. Totowa, N.J.: Rowman and Littlefield.

Ross, Judith, John Glaser, Dorothy Rasinski-Gregory, Joan Gibson, and Corrine Bayley. 1993. *Health Care Ethics Committees: The Next Generation*. Chicago, Ill.: American Hospital Publishing.

Roth, Loren, Alan Meisel, and Charles Lidz. 1977. "Tests of Competency to Consent to Treatment," *American Journal of Psychiatry* 134:279–84.

Rudolph, Wallace. 1966. "The Duty to Act: A Proposed Rule." In James M. Radcliffe (ed.), *The Good Samaritan and the Law*. Garden City, N.Y.: Anchor Books.

Scofield, Giles. 1993. "Ethics Consultation: The Least Dangerous Profession?" *Cambridge Quarterly of Healthcare Ethics* 2, no. 4: 417–26.

Shalit, Ruth. 1997. "When We Were Philosopher Kings," *New Republic* (April 28): 24–28.

Smith, Patricia. 1990. "The Duty to Rescue and the Slippery Slope Problem," *Social Theory and Practice* 16, no. 1: 19–41.

Society for Health and Human Values–Society for Bioethics Consultation, Task Force on Standards for Bioethics Consultation. 1998. *Core Competencies for Health Care Ethics Consultation*. Glenview, Ill.: American Society for Bioethics and Humanities.

Taylor, Telford. 1971. *Nuremberg and Vietnam: An American Tragedy*. New York: Bantam Books.

Tichtchenko, Pavel. 1995. "The Individual and Healthcare in the New Russia," *Cambridge Quarterly of Healthcare Ethics* 4, no. 1: 75–79.

Tollefsen, Christopher. 1998. "Response to 'Reassessing the Reliability of Advance Directives' by Thomas May: Advance Directives and Voluntary Slavery," *Cambridge Quarterly of Healthcare Ethics* 7, no. 4: 405–13.

Turner, Aletha, and the Illinois Guardianship and Advocacy Commission. 1999. "Adult Guardianship in Illinois." In Thomas May and Paul Tudico (eds.), *Advance Directives and Surrogate Decision Making in Illinois*. Springfield, Ill.: Human Services Press.

Waldron, Jeremy. 1981. "A Right to Do Wrong," *Ethics* 92:21–39.

Wear, Stephen. 1998. *Informed Consent: Patient Autonomy and Clinician Beneficence within Health Care*, 2nd ed. Washington, D.C.: Georgetown University Press.

Whelan, John M. 1991. "Charity and the Duty to Rescue," *Social Theory and Practice* 17, no. 3: 441–56.

Winston, Morton, Sally Winston, Paul Appelbaum, and Nancy Rhoden. 1982. "Can a Subject Consent to a 'Ulysses Contract'?" *Hastings Center Report* 12, no. 4 (August): 26–28.

References

Wolf, Susan. 1987. "Sanity and the Metaphysics of Responsibility." In Ferdinand Schoeman (ed.), *Responsibility, Character, and the Emotions*. New York: Cambridge University Press.

INDEX

Index

harm principle, 22–23, 86
Hohfeld, W., 6

indirect strategies, 28–30, 56–63
informed consent, 3, 13–32, 37–39, 95,
106–107, 113; and disclosure, 16–21, 31;
exceptions to, 21–30; international approaches, 3–4; as a partnership, 20–21;
waiver of, 14, 21, 28–30

Jehovah's Witnesses, 16, 25, 47, 99

Kant, Immanuel, 2, 67
Kaplan, Kenneth, 34

law, 38, 43–46, 51–52, 64–66; and health
care, 51–52; as social policy, 38, 43–44,
45–46, 64–66
liberalism, 2–9, 39–40, 47–48, 87, 88–91,
106–107, 110, 123–124
liberty, negative and positive, 6–9
life plans, 3, 67–71
life support, 47, 49, 109–112
living wills, 56, 70, 73–74

Malm, Heidi, 83, 87
mental illness, 25, 43
merit, 33, 44–45
Mill, John Stuart, 2–3, 22, 24, 26, 39, 123
Montefiore, Alan, 115
moral beliefs, 1, 16, 81, 102
moral theory, 2–4, 36

paternalism, 15, 19, 72, 81
personal identity, 55–56
physician-assisted suicide, 98–99
physician-patient relationship, 1, 81, 91–96
practical reasoning, 57–63, 66–71
President's Commission for the Study of
Ethical Problems in Medicine and
Biomedical and Behavioral Research,
33
professional standards, 17–19
prohibitions, vs. requirements, 5–6,
109–113

provider rights of conscience, 9, 82,
99–113, 121; and access to health care,
100–101; in conflict with patient
autonomy, 98–99; and discrimination,
100
public health, 22–23

quality of life, 1, 16, 71, 107, 109

Rawls, John, 2, 3, 67–68, 87
Raz, Joseph, 22–23, 28–30, 57–63, 65, 69
reasonable person standard, 19–20
requests, vs. refusals, 109–113
responsibility, 40–41, 45–46
rights, 3, 5–9, 82; negative, 6–9, 90; positive, 6–9
Rudolph, Wallace, 85

Sandel, Michael, 67
sanity, 43, 39–47; and autonomy, 39–47
Scofield, Giles, 118, 122–125
second-order reasoning, 28–30, 57–70,
90–91
self, 41, 55–56
Shalit, Ruth, 118–120
Smith, Patricia, 84
subjectivity, 19, 20–21
substituted judgment, 50–52
surrogate decision making, 3, 51–52,
75–76

Task Force on Standards for Bioethics
Consultation (SHHV-SBC), 117, 122
technology, 1, 15
therapeutic privilege, 21, 26–30
toleration, 3, 81, 100, 115
Tollefsen, Christopher, 63–71
transfer of care, 99–100, 104
treatment: alternatives, 13, 15–16; determining appropriateness of, 1, 9, 22,
105–107, 110, 119–121
trust, 30
type, 33, 44–45, 102–107, 112–113

utilitarianism, 2–3

Index

values, 1–3, 14–16, 19–21, 34, 99–100,
107–108; imposition of, 1, 15; individual, 1, 2, 14–16, 19–21, 107; religious, 16,
99–100, 108; role of, 1, 14–15, 19–20, 107
voluntary slavery, 61–62

vulnerability, 37, 104, 115

well-being, 34, 36–38, 90, 107
Whelan, John, 84–85
Wolf, Susan, 41–42